Women, Health, and Poverty

Women, Health, and Poverty

Cesar A. Perales, LLB
Lauren S. Young, EdD
Editors

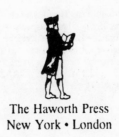

The Haworth Press
New York • London

Women, Health, and Poverty has also been published as *Women & Health*, Volume 12, Numbers 3/4, 1987.

The Haworth Press, Inc., 12 West 32 Street, New York, NY 10001
EUROSPAN/Haworth, 3 Henrietta Street, London WC2E 8LU England

Library of Congress Cataloging-in-Publication Data

Women, health, and poverty.

   (Women & health ; v. 12, no. 3/4)
   Includes bibliographies.
   1. Women — Economic conditions — Health aspects — United States.
2. Minorities — Economic conditions — Health aspects — United States. 3. Poverty — Health aspects — United States. 4. Women — Health and hygiene — United States.
5. Minorities — Health and hygiene — United States. I. Perales, Cesar A., 1940- .
II. Young, Lauren S. III. Series.
RG1.W64   vol. 12, no. 3/4   362.1'088042 s   87-26274
[RA564.85]   [362.1'088042]
ISBN 0-86656-684-8

Women, Health, and Poverty

CONTENTS

ABOUT THE EDITORS

Cesar A. Perales was appointed Commissioner of New York State's Department of Social Services by Governor Mario Cuomo on February 1, 1983. As administrator of the department, he is responsible for all public assistance programs, Medicaid, child support enforcement, disability determination, adult homes, child protective services, foster care, adoption, and many other programs that help the vulnerable. Mr. Perales came to the department from the Puerto Rican Legal Defense and Education Fund where he had served as President and General Counsel. One of its founders, he was the organization's first Chief Executive. Mr. Perales served under President Jimmy Carter as Assistant Secretary for Human Development Services, the social services branch of the U.S. Department of Health and Human Services. A member of the New York State Bar, he is a graduate of City College of New York and Fordham University School of Law.

Lauren S. Young received her EdD from the Department of Administration, Planning, and Social Policy at Harvard University in 1984. Her research into how social policies affect the education of poor children, particularly in urban schools, is continuing at Michigan State University where she is currently Assistant Professor in the Department of Teacher Education. She is working with the Holmes Group and the National Center for Research on Teacher Education and teaches a course entitled "School and Society." Dr. Young was previously a special assistant to Commissioner Cesar A. Perales in New York State's Department of Social Services where she collaborated in analyzing and formulating social policies to improve services to poor children and families.

Acknowledgement

The papers in this volume were written by invited participants to a roundtable symposium "Women, Poverty and Health: An Analysis and Agenda for the Future," convened by Cesar A. Perales, New York State Commissioner of Social Services, on November 18, 1986 in Albany, New York. Judith Berek, Deputy Commissioner for Adult Services, Lauren S. Young, Special Assistant to the Commissioner and Jeanne Mager Stellman, Editor of *Women & Health*, provided major input in the conceptualization and actualization of the symposium.

Preface

INTRODUCTION

Despite three decades of dramatic social change, adult women—regardless of race or ethnicity, urban or rural residency, age or labor force participation—are more likely than men to be poor. Events experienced by millions each year—divorce, chronic illness, job-related injuries, low-wage occupations, out-of-wedlock child-bearing, retirement, loss of income on the death of a spouse—contribute to the alarming number of women in poverty and the deepening extent of their impoverishment.

Although we have made progress in broadening opportunities for self-sufficiency and in improving the quality of services, we cannot rest on past achievements. Much work remains on behalf of all segments of our client population. This special issue of *Women & Health* takes a hard look at the well-being of poor women in North America. It provides a rare opportunity to focus on one of the most pressing, but neglected social issues of our time—the injurious health consequences of impoverishment among women.

With a continued commitment to compassionate and efficient social services programs, I have called together this distinguished group of experts to review the adequacy of our social and health policies. Each author brings a different voice and style, in some cases deviating from an academic inquiry and presentation. I have welcomed this diversity and introspection. Enhanced by such varied backgrounds and experience, their commentaries on a wide range of issues portray telling accounts of the dynamic interface of poverty, gender, and health and the merits of federal and state efforts.

THE ISSUES

The diversity in the population of poor women is a major topic underscored throughout this volume. It is a significant theme in Dr. Julie Boatright Wilson's overview of poor women in this country. Wilson reviews census data for the twenty-five-year period from 1959 to 1984 and reports that for every year, the poverty rate for women has been consistently higher than that for men, and once poor, women remain in poverty for longer periods of time than men. Describing various paths to poverty, she explains why these events have such devastating effects on women. Wilson rejects single-focus, unidimensional policies for alleviating poverty as "quick-fix" solutions stemming from stereotypical images of poor women. More responsive government policies, she advises, must address the wide variance in the population of this nation's poor women.

Dr. Hila Richardson also writes of the diversity in the population of poor women. While she reports health-risk increases as income decreases independent of place of residence, Richardson's focus is on the well-being of poor women in nonmetropolitan areas. A host of factors such as lack of transportation, isolation from a range of health care resources, and shortages of health care personnel, emergency services, and hospital beds place additional burdens on access to quality health care in rural environments.

Characteristics of rural life — limited opportunities for part-time employment, employer insurance plans, adult education, job-training programs, and child-care facilities, for example — make it even more difficult for poor rural women to overcome their poverty status. Medicaid and Medicare eligibility criteria and program biases against rural poor residents compound the dilemma. For those dependent on public support, the more conservative nature of local governments in rural areas as well as the smaller tax base of rural communities, Richardson informs us, result in public assistance programs with fewer benefits and services.

Another characteristic marking the diversity of poor women is their labor force participation. Working full-time in one of several occupations can mean a life of poverty for a woman and her family. In her review of 1980 census data, Dr. Jeanne M. Stellman shows that the majority of women workers in this country are in occupations in which at least 10 percent of all full-time employed women workers are impoverished. And, depending on the industry, age, and race/ethnicity of the female worker, the proportions in poverty can rise significantly. In building services and laundry-work jobs, for example, 28 to 43 percent of unmarried nonwhite women under the age of 45 who work full-time had incomes at or below the poverty level. Yet, while higher proportions of impoverished, full-time employed women workers are concentrated in some industries, Stellman tells us that they can also be found among clerical and office workers, industrial and agricultural workers, and workers in the service industries.

Despite the early passage of laws in this country to protect female workers, impoverished women are typically employed in industries that present grave risks to their health and safety brought by occupational exposures, high stress levels, adverse working conditions, and insufficient attention to these conditions. Drawing on workers' compensation data, one of the few sources of quantitative data on job injuries and illnesses, Stellman describes the health and safety conditions of the work environments of working-poor women. Despite the dearth of data available on women workers, she estimates that 250,000 female, full-time workers holding jobs in occupations employing significant numbers of impoverished or poverty-stricken workers were seriously enough injured or disabled on the job to file a claim with their state workers' compensation system in 1980. The physical demands and a number of toxins and other dangerous conditions present in the work environments in occupations that pay low wages leave working-poor women at risk for developing occupational-related maladies and injuries.

An environment of poverty typically presents health hazards in other areas of women's lives. Poverty as a major health problem is a predominate theme in the discussion by Ms. Lorna McBarnette, who reviews the effects of poverty on reproductive status. Citing evidence from New York State, the nation, and other countries, McBarnette documents a variety of physical health conditions brought by impoverishment. Data on the utilization of family-planning and prenatal-care services, complications associated with sexually transmitted diseases, maternal death, nutrition, and incidences of cervical cancer all show that poor women are significantly worse off in comparison with women of higher economic status. In fact, as socioeconomic status declines, McBarnette argues, so do indices of positive health status.

McBarnette attributes the differences in the reproductive well-being of poor and nonpoor women in the United States to disparities in the financial and other resources available to pay for health and medical care. For women who are poor, access to such care is lacking and deficient, and with long-term health consequences. While Medicaid is the public health program for the poor, McBarnette reports that less than 40 percent of the population with incomes below the poverty level were covered by Medicaid in 1980. Nor does enrollment in the Medicaid program guarantee access to health care. The number of obstetricians and gynecologists who provide specialized reproductive care and participate in the Medicaid program, or treat uninsured women, is decreasing. Four of ten physicians who provided obstetrical and gynecological care in 1985, McBarnette reports, did not accept Medicaid clients. She calls for a new ideological commitment and state responsibility for a comprehensive health services system that ensures access to quality health care for all women, regardless of socioeconomic status and age.

Risks for ill-health are not limited to physical well-being. Several of the papers provide rich accounts of the debilitating effects of impoverishment on women's mental health. Dr. Maisha B. H. Bennett shares case-study vignettes in her essay on the experiences of Afro-American poor women to illustrate poverty as a state of mind and as a risk factor for mental illness. While the U.S. Bureau of the Census definition is the common measure of poverty, Bennett suggests additional standards for appraising impoverishment: the relativity of poverty, transient vs. chronic poverty, and first generational vs. intergenerational poverty. Expanding opportunities for employment and reshaping public assistance programs to reinforce family stability and the presence of fathers and husbands figure prominently among her recommendations.

In framing our policies, Bennett informs us, policymakers also must take into account the number of poor women whose responses to poverty-induced stresses include a number of emotional and psychological disorders as well as alcohol and other substance dependencies. Public mental health promotions and education campaigns directed toward changing attitudes and modifying behaviors of the poor at all stages of the life cycle are strategies she recommends as part of progressive social reform.

Ms. Freda L. Paltiel adds an international context and perspective to the discussion of poverty, gender, and mental health. As in the United States, Canadian women are overrepresented among the poor. Paltiel's comprehensive review of the salient literature on stress, coping, and mental health among poor women, including studies emanating from the International Women's decade, support a major theme: women are overworked and undervalued throughout the world, and the relationship between women's work and women's worth has profound consequences for their mental health.

Paltiel proposes a three-anchor needs framework of work, family, and friendship and a coping schema to provide direction and guidance for self-understanding and for helping poor women to acquire the resources, supports, attributes, and perspectives to better cope with the effects of poverty on mental health. She recommends that research and policies formulated on a hierarchy of human needs and on a goal of self-actualization be replaced with the coping schema presented as a potentially more effective mediator of stressors brought by social condition.

The discussion provided by Dr. Carlota Texidor del Portillo centers on the unique at-risk group of Latino women who underutilize mental health services and are prone to be misdiagnosed and mistreated. Providing demographic and socioeconomic overviews of Latinos/Hispanics in the United States, del Portillo raises concerns about the limited research literature and scarce epidemiological data on the physical and mental well-being of Hispanics/Latinos, immigrants and descendants from more than 30 countries in which the Spanish language is spoken. Del Portillo argues throughout for better data-collection efforts and for information disaggregated beyond the three major Hispanic groups in the U.S.: Mexican-Americans, Puerto Ricans, and Cubans, efforts that would better enable agencies to develop programs and refine services for members of the diverse groups that make up this population.

Del Portillo prescribes a vocational and counseling approach used at San Francisco Mission Community College for its effectiveness among Latino women. In designing counseling, mental health programs, and other intervention strategies, she recommends therapies tailored from a psychology of development and individual differences rather than from a psychology of adjustment.

Special issues facing poor women of color is the topic of the essay by Dr. Ruth Gordon-Bradshaw. That poor women of color are subjected to minority status and to inequitable practices stemming from racism, discrimination, and sexism is a predominant theme. By reviewing selected indicators in education, living environment, employment and income, and health, Gordon-Bradshaw argues that racial, gender, and class biases in U.S. society underlie the impoverished state of many women of color, and the difficulty they face in trying to overcome their poverty. She posits several recommendations, both for policymakers and for women of color.

Just as poverty bears heavily on the health of the poor, poor health can propel others to indigence. Catastrophic illnesses, chronic health conditions, and the inadequacies of public health insurance programs are key factors that drive many into poverty. While these events affect all but the very wealthy, they are particularly catastrophic for the elderly, and especially elderly women.

Dr. Lois Grau draws our attention to the elderly poor and to the significant number of persons who enter old age with incomes near the poverty level who become impoverished during the course of aging. Because gender differences in longevity result in a larger ratio of females to males as we age and because women are more likely to experience multiple, chronic, and increasingly debilitating diseases prior to death, Grau argues that the consequences of a long-term illness and debilitation are particularly catastrophic for elderly women.

While we have witnessed significant advances in alleviating poverty among the elderly over the last two decades, Grau reminds us that poverty and poor health is a two-way condition. A chronic illness among the nonpoor can precipitate impoverishment as a result of public policies that require individuals to spend down to poverty levels, to divest resources, and other eligibility criteria for publicly supported health and social programs. Although Medicaid is an important safety net for the elderly poor, as is Medicare, the assistance these programs provide does not go far enough in meeting their health care needs. Grau argues for experimenting with various types of long-term care insurance, shifting from costly hospital-based and nursing-home care to comprehensive community-based services, and expanding Medicare benefits to better meet the long-term-care and other health care needs of older individuals.

New York State Assemblyman James R. Tallon and Ms. Rachel Block in their discussion of health insurance coverage highlight similar strengths and failures of the public health care system. Where Grau focuses solely on the special vulnerability of older women, Tallon and Block show that despite dramatic increases in health care expenditures and utilization in recent years, an erosion of insurance coverage has created gaps in services to the elderly and also to other segments of the population. With most group insurance tied to full-time participation in the labor force and less likely provided in the types of industries and job sectors where most women are employed, women of all ages are especially at risk.

Millions of Americans are forced to forego medical insurance for themselves and their families because they are unable to afford individual medical policies. Others lose their health insurance when they lose their spouse through death or divorce. Still others, Tallon and Block argue, face significant gaps in health care coverage as a result of Medicaid spend-down policies and the failure of the Medicare program—where 60 percent of the enrollees are women—to cover various major health care expenses of the elderly. From this vantage, Tallon and Block recommend a comprehensive approach to ensure universal access to health care.

Dr. Shirley L. Zimmerman draws upon exchange and choice theories to set the context for her study of state-level policy as a predictor of individual and family well-being. Using 1980 state per capita expenditures for education, health, public welfare as measures of state policy, Zimmerman examines the relationship of these state spending patterns to indices of individual and family well-being or social malaise: suicide, rates of infant death, and teenage birthrates.

Zimmerman's findings show that higher state expenditures for public welfare and education are positive predictors of individual and family well-being as measured by lower state rates of suicide and teenage births. Conversely, states that spend less show higher teenage birthrates, infant deaths, and suicides. Zimmerman suggests that these findings highlight the central importance of education, income adequacy, and security for individual and family well-being, and the critical role that state-level public policy can play. Her findings compel us to explore further the meanings of these relationships. Given the diminishing role of the federal government in human affairs since 1980, her recommendations are particularly timely.

Another major theme in this volume centers on the failures and limited explanatory power of past research models, analyses, and data on the interrelationship of gender, class, and race/ethnicity. While some improvements in national data collection have been made, the gaps that remain and the manner in which local health statistics are maintained often preclude the ability to analyze these data for inferences about women. Although the needs of women have garnered much public attention over the last two decades, the research has not kept pace with the need for better understanding the context, health, utilization patterns, health practices, and help-seeking behaviors of different cohorts of poor and racial/ethnic women. Dr. Ruth E. Zambrana seeks to bridge this void by positing a research agenda and model for better information-gathering.

Zambrana's research agenda arises from the incomplete research and knowledge about factors that influence health conditions among poor and racial/ethnic women, and emphasizes selected substantive areas: reproductive health, health practice, poor and racial/ethnic minority women, and aging, and the relationship between chronic life stress, social support, and health status and functioning. Focusing on each of these factors unveils a variety of other issues related to socioeconomic status that influence women's health. She reminds us of the plurality and interactive nature of these factors, suggesting that they cannot be fully understood outside the contexts in which they arise. The formulation of a more encompassing model and research agenda, Zambrana advises, may be an important first step in improving the quality of life of low-income and racial/ethnic women.

PRESENT DIRECTIONS

The unavailability and limited access to quality and affordable health care aggravate an already unsettling situation for women in poverty. Because the basis of women's health plight is often their poverty, economic, social, and health policy responses share importance.

The findings and experiences presented in this publication show that one avenue for improving the health status of poor women is to provide ways for helping them to overcome their poverty. Throughout this nation, states have taken the initiative to confront this important problem. I am proud that we in New York in the last four years have taken aggressive and creative steps in a number of arenas. Our actions have been not only to ensure that the social services system supports those who need it, but that it also provides those who seek a way out of poverty an opportunity to reach those dreams.

The mission of the state Department of Social Services is to ensure that dependent and disabled persons in New York State, those whose incomes are insufficient to provide the bare necessities for living for themselves and their families, receive the financial, medical, and other supportive services necessary to achieve the greatest amount of independence. As we enter the second term of Governor Mario M. Cuomo's administration, and the fifth year of our leadership of the New York State Department of Social Services, we can point to significant accomplishments both in broadening opportunities for self-sufficiency and in improving the quality of services for those who remain dependent.

Adequate Child Support Awards and Enforcement

Adequate levels of child support and enforcement of child support awards can be an effective strategy for helping many women avoid poverty. Increased authority and practices to carry out these activities are the result in part of the changing role of welfare support for families. When the national welfare program was created in 1935 as Aid to Dependent Children (ADC), it essentially was to provide long-term income support for widowed mothers. A woman was not expected to seek or to be able to earn an income for herself and for her children. It was not until the 1950s, as divorce became more common, that children with living fathers were represented significantly in the ADC caseload. Even then, however, absent fathers were assumed outside the purview of federal relief, both in eligibility and, largely, in responsibility.

Vestiges of these outmoded assumptions remain. While mothers are the custodial parent in the vast majority of divorces and separations, child support accounts for only 10 percent of the income of female-headed households, even given the expanded child-support activities made possible by Title IV-D of the Social Security Act. Only a small minority of children on Aid to Families with Dependent Children (AFDC) receive support from their fathers, although some 90 percent of these children have living fathers.

We have had some success in altering these dynamics, and in reframing the assumptions and expections of AFDC. With better management tools, more efficient administration, and strengthened child support enforcement authority, this state has put forth a concerted effort to supplement the incomes of parents in custody of children who are threatened with the need for or must rely on public assistance resulting from divorce and loss of income in the support of their children. Our activities have produced steadily increasing child support collections, both for AFDC and non-AFDC custodial parents over the last several years. In fact, total collections rose 41 percent between 1981 and 1985, going from $145 million to $204 million. These efforts are part of an overall strategy to strengthen the ability of families to remain or become independent, and at the same time underscore the importance of parental responsibility in the support of families.

Employment and Training Opportunities

AFDC, founded on the antiquated notion that a mother's only role is caring for her children at home, is being transformed in the employment arena as well. Like the majority of American women with children today, public assistance clients want to work and would willingly take a job if one were available at their level of skills. The problems are that fewer such jobs are available, that these jobs are at low wages, and that they typically provide no family health insurance coverage.

Understanding that job services and training opportunities are part of the foundation for enabling families to become self-sufficient, New York State has pioneered the development of employment programs, enlisting the individual services our clients need to help them find a job. Like other states, New York is pushing forward with initiatives making available such services as employability assessments, training, job-placement services, and a variety of support services to strengthen an individual's ability to secure employment. Public welfare clients are now being offered more intensive training and employment programs, whether it means completion of a high school education, developing confidence, on-the-job training, or actual work experience. We have cooperated with employers and relied on part of the welfare check as a subsidy to train individuals for specific jobs in the private sector. We have initiated projects at several community colleges so that AFDC mothers can develop the skills needed by industry. By providing adequate child care and an array of other support services, education, and training opportunities, our new Comprehensive Employment Opportunity Support Centers will soon be models of what can be done for women with young children. I see these efforts as government at its best, making investments in people who can and want to become self-sufficient, but who need some help along the way.

Special efforts must also be made to provide intensive services for young women, who are most in danger of becoming long-term dependents on public assistance. Faced with the tragedy of children bearing children, we have moved forward with a comprehensive approach to adolescent pregnancy. Governor Cuomo's Avenues to Dignity program offers young people parenting and job-training programs, education support, and health and child care services to reduce unwanted teen pregnancy. Various teenage pregnancy case management projects are other examples of our attempts to reshape the public welfare system by assigning a case manager to each young mother in these projects in an attempt to provide the individual attention and to coordinate the needed services to assist these young women. We want to ensure that all these young people also have opportunities for advancement.

Understanding the necessity of accessible and affordable day care for working parents and for parents who seek employment, we have expanded the availability of family and community-based day care in communities throughout the state. "Latchkey children" and their parents are being provided an alternative to unsupervised activities by funding to develop community child-care programs. We have established pilot Child Development Center programs, all with the intent of extending recruitment of family day-care providers. At the same time, we are pushing forward to increase the number of licensed family day-care providers. We also have funded local district projects, expanding day care to support training and employment for public assistance and low-income families who were negatively affected by federal cuts in income-eligible day care and changes in the AFDC program. And, the state has funded day care for the working poor so that they will be able to remain in the workplace and at the same time feel confident that their children are safe.

Yet, New York's response to joblessness, like that of other states, must be a multifaceted approach of innovation and economic development. At the same time that we prepare public assistance clients for the workforce, attention must also be focused on the demand side of the employment equation. The most effective training and job-placement programs will not work unless there are jobs. The development of economic employment zones in various economically depressed areas across the state should serve as a good beginning. The federal government shares responsibility, too. With increases in real wages linked closely to decreases in the poverty rate, economic growth is a key component of an effective anti-poverty effort. National strategies supportive of a strong, productive, and high-employment economy; wage levels that can support individuals and families above the poverty level; and assurances of antidiscriminatory and equitable practices in hiring and wages are fundamental and necessary as well.

Adequate Benefit Levels

Providing for the dependent is an unnegotiable responsibility of the social services system. Differences among states in benefit levels, however, point to glaring inequities in the public assistance system. How well one can provide the basic necessities for living is dependent partly on where one resides. For a family of three, for example, monthly benefits range from $740 in Alaska to $497 in New York City to $302 in Ohio to $120 in Mississippi.

New York has been a leader among states in advocating for adequate benefit levels to enable families to purchase the basic essentials for living. In January 1984, we were able to raise the public assistance shelter allowance by an average of 25 percent throughout New York State, the first increase to reflect changes in the relative rent levels since the shelter allowance maximums were first set in 1975. We also secured a 10 percent home energy allowance increase to the basic needs standard, effective January 1, 1986, the first increase of its kind since 1981. These gains undoubtedly benefit the condition of low-income New Yorkers by improving access to housing and by providing an increase in much-needed dispensable income.

Yet, in almost every state in 1986, public assistance benefits, including Food Stamps, do not amount to the poverty level. The median state AFDC benefit of $346 per month and $178 per month in Food Stamps amount to only $6,288 per year, just 73 percent of the poverty level for a family of three. It is not hard to see that much remains to be done.

Food Stamps and Nutrition

The positive link between nutrition and health is well-established. Passage of state nutrition education legislation in 1984 has allowed the department to increase public awareness of the importance of good nutrition, the availability of Food Stamps and nutrition education services, and ways of getting the most from food dollars. The goal of our nutrition education campaign is to promote wiser use of more than $900 million in Food Stamps distributed in New York State.

States have acted decisively to protect Food Stamp benefits threatened by federal cuts. One of the major dilemmas arises from states' efforts to ensure adequate public assistance benefit levels and the subsequent effects on Food Stamp allotments. U.S. Department of Agriculture (USDA) regulations now require that any increases in public assistance benefits be counted as income when the Food Stamp allotment is determined. Thus for every $3 increase in public assistance, Food Stamp benefits to the same household are reduced by $1.

Although we have been unsuccessful thus far in turning around this federal ruling, New York has worked closely with other states to increase benefits to counteract these reductions in Food Stamps. For example, in reaction to raising the portion of the state grant allotted for shelter in 1984, USDA directed the state to reduce Food Stamps accordingly. Working with members of Congress, and with Congressman Leon Panetta's leadership as chair of the House Subcommittee on Food Stamps, we were successful in lobbying Congress to increase Food Stamp benefits from 99 percent to 100 percent of the Thrifty Food Plan, an increase shared by Food Stamp recipients across the country. While this increase did not totally offset the loss of benefits to clients, it substantially alleviated the problem.

Fairer Standards for Disability Determinations

The Office of Disability Determinations is the New York State agency responsible for adjudicating medical eligibility for the state's disabled population under Titles II and XVI of the Social Security Act. New York State has been in the forefront of the fight against the federal government's restrictive disability reviews.

In July 1983, New York State triggered a nationwide rebellion against the federal disability program when I refused to continue the massive and arbitrary removal of New York's Title II disability recipients — 32 percent of primary beneficiaries who are women — from Social Security rolls until the federal government developed a reasonable medical improvement standard by which disability benefits could be reviewed fairly and uniformly. States were being forced by the federal government to cut off the benefits of these individuals even though they may not have shown any physical or mental improvement since qualifying for disability payments. This moratorium, the first of its kind in any state, was just one of several steps taken to force a change in federal policy that resulted in the wholesale denial and termination of benefits to thousands of disabled people, including more than 25,000 individuals in New York State alone.

New York sought redress in the courts and took its battle for the rights of the physically and mentally disabled to Congress, where legislation passed that included provisions for which New York State had been advocating. We will continue to monitor disability determination criteria in our resolve to ensure fair and equitable practices.

Services to Victims of Domestic Violence

With growing recognition of spousal abuse as a major national social problem, we have devoted considerable energy and resources to developing shelters for those who require safe, temporary refuge. While domestic violence is in no way limited to the poor, these individuals often do not have the resources to move out of abusive circumstances. Over the last three years, more than $1.5 million, including funds provided by the federal Family Violence Prevention and Services Act, has supported domestic violence programs statewide to provide shelter and supportive services for abused spouses and their children. We have contracted with the New York State Coalition Against Domestic Violence to manage a bilingual (English/Spanish) hotline for victims of domestic violence. We have also developed outreach, advocacy, and counseling services for victims of domestic violence in rural areas of New York State, where no services had existed, and in underserved communities in urban areas. States are just beginning to understand the parameters of this problem. We will need to oversee an extension of services as the demand for safe shelter increases.

Health Care for the Poor

We also understand that the goal of independence and dignity cannot be addressed by income maintenance and employment programs alone. Society and government must also address the issues of affordable, accessible, and available health care, a major theme highlighted throughout this volume.

The Medicaid program, enacted in 1965 by an amendment to the Social Security Act, provides a broad range of health care benefits to poor, eligible individuals. There is no doubt that the program has greatly increased the amount of health care that poor people receive, and has gone a long way toward closing the gap between rich and poor in terms of access to and use of health care. Yet, despite substantial annual investments in health care for the poor, problems remain. A significant portion of poor individuals are not eligible for the program; those who are enrolled are more likely than the non-Medicaid population to receive fragmented and episodic care in high cost settings; and steady, preventive health care is still far from the norm.

The problem is based partly in the structure of the Medicaid program and New York State has undertaken the job of reforming it. We have advocated strongly for alternatives to the fee-for-service reimbursement system, which has fostered an undesirable reliance on care provided in hospital emergency rooms and outpatient departments. We are making strides in improved access to quality and continuity of care, particularly preventive health care, through the Child/Teen Health Plan and by promoting Medicaid client enrollment in health maintenance organizations (HMOs) or similar programs.

We see HMOs as a means for providing poor families the opportunities to participate in comprehensive, prepaid health plans, and to receive coordinated, supervised primary care. Medicap, an innovative project in New York's Monroe County, is a unique, prepaid health plan demonstration and one example of the state's efforts in Medicaid reform. The program involves all of the county's welfare recipients selecting health providers associated with HMOs. More than 40,000 recipients, or virtually all those eligible for AFDC and Home Relief cash assistance in Monroe County, have been enrolled. The outcome of this experiment in managed care, the largest of its kind in the United States, will have a bearing on the way health care is provided for the needy in New York State and across the nation.

As is the case nationally, longer life spans, the high cost of medical care, and the rapidly growing population of elderly citizens are extending the demands on state-supported health and supportive services. For example, while the elderly comprise less than 10 percent of New York's Medicaid population, more than 50 percent of Medicaid dollars is spent on care for the elderly and the chronically ill. Long-term custodial care and outpatient prescription drugs, which are important and costly services for many elderly persons, are ineligible for reimbursement under Medicare. The implication of these figures and policies on the state's long-term care system are great, especially for the Medicaid program, which currently finances the major share of these services. Given its key role, the financing of such services will continue to exert greater pressure on states' fiscal resources.

Nursing-home care places enormous financial strain on the elderly and their families. While some individuals require the supervision and services provided in these settings, most older adults prefer to stay at home and could remain independent if support services were available. To help address this need, in 1983 a number of counties in New York State began a locally-based program, Community Alternative Systems Agencies, to match the needs of these individuals with appropriate care. This program has not only resulted in better placements for the elderly, but it also has reduced hospital stays and saved taxpayers' dollars.

An innovative program for long-term care being tested in New York State also will help assure improved access to community-based services. Known as the "Nursing Home Without Walls," this program is designed to provide an alternative to institutional care for the chronically ill, the disabled, and the infirm elderly. Through close case management and patient monitoring, and by drawing upon family, community, voluntary, and other informal support services networks, the program provides a comprehensive set of health, social, and environmental services to patients while they live at home. Already, this system has reduced the length of time elderly patients must wait in hospitals for placements in the community.

New York State also helps older adults to remain independent by providing a range of services in their communities, including personal care, protective services, and long-term home health care. To ensure low-cost alternatives to nursing homes, this past year we strengthened the nation's largest community-based residential care system by increasing the amount of money the state provides to help the elderly live in these homes. There are approximately 60,000 recipients of home care in New York State, more recipients than in any other state receiving such care. Like other reforms instituted by the department in the last four years, these services allow both the elderly and nonelderly to remain in their homes or in community-based settings.

The demand for long-term health care services is swelling and will continue to intensify through the end of this century. Health and human services policymakers across the country will need to reevaluate current policies and programs, as well as develop creative solutions that address these evolving needs.

AN AGENDA FOR THE FUTURE

I believe that over the last four years we in New York State, like the administrations in many states, have laid the important groundwork for attending to the needs and concerns described so eloquently in this volume. We recognize the complexity of these growing problems and understand that the response to these issues must be a multifaceted one. We also understand that present federal policy that assigns to states responsibility for these solutions ignores important factors. It ignores that the elderly and the poor are not evenly distributed among states. It ignores that poverty in this country in part stems from federal policies. It inequitably asks those with a smaller tax base and with little voice in macroeconomic and national decisions to take responsibility for the products of those policies. Since 1981, the human services have borne the brunt of federal austerity. These authors remind us of the severe consequences shared by all members of society when we ignore the less fortunate and those who have fallen on bad times. We must continue to move forward.

Attending to the mandate of an accessible, quality, and affordable health care system requires a more comprehensive strategy to prevention, services, and financing than that provided by the course of current federal and state programs. Far greater focus on prevention and primary care services would help alleviate many of the conditions described herein. More attention to the interactive effects of poverty, gender, and the ecology of living and work environments would address others. The key issue centers around state and federal policymakers conceptualizing a more dynamic model of public health care. That is, a more effective and efficient approach to public health would emphasize and focus on environmental conditions—housing, nutrition, safe work environments, prenatal care, for example—that influence health status just as it should ensure that quality health care is accessible, available, and affordable. With such a direction and commitment, a more coherent and coordinated health care policy and a better health care system is possible.

In effect, our task is to frame a social policy agenda that more effectively and efficiently responds to the socioeconomic dilemmas of the poor in general and of poor women in particular. In order to better develop this agenda, the authors tell us that better data and data-collection efforts are needed. We can no longer afford to ignore the diversity in the demography and characteristics of those who are poor. The limited data available on women and more specifically poor women call for federal, state, and local governments and agencies to extend the groups on whom data are collected such that we have better information and analyses from which to formulate policy.

Our policies must begin to pay closer attention to gaps in medical coverage and to the pressing concerns of working-poor families and those with incomes near the poverty level who are unable to afford health insurance or medical care. Because Medicaid eligibility is limited largely to public assistance eligibility, millions of families in and near poverty are left uninsured. It is important to establish the medical assistance eligibility standard at a level that will protect working-poor and poor two-parent families and that will ease the transition of other families from public assistance to employment.

Our agenda must begin by sharing responsibility for the millions of Americans who are sustained but not fundamentally helped by social and health policies. It must provide a way to respond meaningfully and expressively to the social, economic, and health needs of indigent individuals and families. It must restore hope to impoverished families, not only in New York State, but across the country. And it cannot end until our national government, like us, recognizes that poverty in America is an estrangement that we can no longer ignore. The consequences on the health and well-being of this nation and that of future generations are far too great.

Cesar A. Perales
Commissioner
New York State Department of Social Services

Women and Poverty:
A Demographic Overview

Julie Boatright Wilson, PhD

SUMMARY. In the current debate about causes and cures for poverty, much attention is given to women. Women are more likely than men to be poor, and once impoverished, to remain poor for longer periods of time than do men. In addition, a much greater responsibility for raising the next generation of adults belongs to poor women than to poor men. No individual policy response will alleviate poverty among women. Rather, a multi-faceted policy response that recognizes the wide diversity of their situations is necessary. This paper describes the diversity among poor women and suggests a series of appropriate policies.

In the current debate about the causes and most appropriate cures for poverty, much has been made of the disproportionate share of misfortune experienced by women. Women are more likely than men to be poor, more likely to remain poor once they enter poverty, and increasingly likely to be left with the responsibility for children without access to the resources of the other parent.

All too often, however, the voices we hear offer stereotypical descriptions of poor women in their rationales for "quick-fix" solutions. By ignoring the diversity in the population of poor women and the changes in this population over time policy makers and others fail to develop and advocate for policies that address the needs of all types of poor women. This paper begins with an examination of the characteristics of poor women and

Julie Boatright Wilson is Director, Office of Program Planning, Analysis and Development, New York State Department of Social Services, 40 North Pearl Street, Albany, NY 12243.

concludes with policy suggestions that address the diversity of their needs.

DEFINING POVERTY

Before presenting characteristics of poor women and discussing the reasons for their poverty, it is useful to define poverty. In the early 1960s, the Social Security Administration developed a definition of poverty based on family size, basic nutritional requirements, the cost of food, and the proportion of household income the typical family spent on food. The basis of the measurement was the U.S. Agriculture Department's "economy food plan," which determined the amount and types of food families of various sizes needed to survive. The cost of purchasing that "market basket" of food was calculated and the poverty level was determined by multiplying this dollar amount by three, since an earlier study had shown that the typical family spent one-third of its income for food. Households with incomes below that level were considered "poor"; households with incomes above that level were considered "not poor."

Since that time the definition of poverty has evolved somewhat. Most important, instead of repricing the "market basket each year," the poverty level of the previous year is updated by the value of the consumer price index. Today's poverty level, however, still reflects the earlier relationship established between poverty and household size, the cost of food, and the proportion of household income devoted to food. And despite the growth in in-kind benefits such as Food Stamps and Medicaid, the poverty rate is still determined on the basis of cash income only.

Table 1 shows the 1985 poverty levels for households of different sizes. To put this in perspective, the median household income is also shown.

Throughout the 1960s, considerable progress was made toward reducing the number of people living in poverty in the United States. But as Figure 1 shows, the proportion of the population with income below the poverty level remained relatively constant throughout the seventies. After 1979, the proportion of the population with income below the poverty level increased, until 1983, when it began declining.

Table 1

1985 Poverty Levels and Median Household Income

Number of Persons in Household	2	3	4	5
Poverty level	$7,420	$8,580	$11,000	$13,030
Median Household Income	23,132	29,265	32,777	31,794

In 1984, the most recent year for which complete data are available, 14.4 percent of the population, or 33.7 million people, lived in households with income below the poverty level. Of these 33.7 million people, 67 percent lived in households with income under 75 percent of the poverty level and 38 percent lived in households with income less than half the poverty level.

WHO ARE THE POOR WOMEN?

The right-hand side of Figure 1 shows the poverty rates for men and women 15 years old and over for the last several years. The lines are approximately parallel. The poverty rate for women, however, is higher in every year than the corresponding poverty rate for men.

The major determinant of women's higher poverty rates appears to be household status. Women who head their own households are nearly five times as likely to be poor as men who head their own households. The data in Table 2, which compare male and female poverty rates across various demographic categories, suggest that while women have higher poverty rates than men in almost every category examined, the patterns of poverty for men and women are similar. For both groups, younger adults, non-whites, those with less than a high school education, those that are not married and those that have periods of unemployment during the year have the highest poverty rates.

Household status appears to be driving the overall higher poverty rates of women. Women who head their own households are

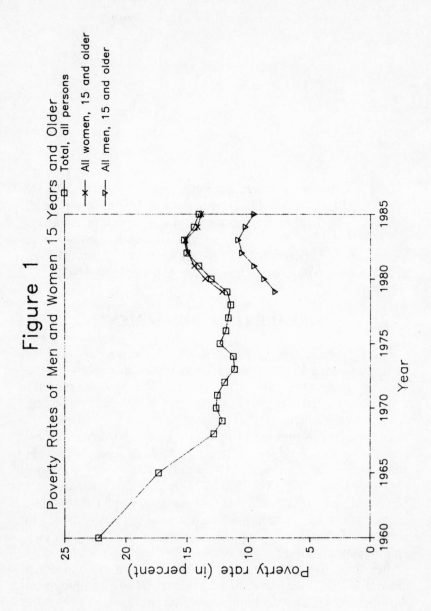

Figure 1

Poverty Rates of Men and Women 15 Years and Older

Legend:
- Total, all persons
- All women, 15 and older
- All men, 15 and older

X-axis: Year (1960, 1965, 1970, 1975, 1980, 1985)

Y-axis: Poverty rate (in percent) (0, 5, 10, 15, 20, 25)

Table 2

Percentage Distribution of Poor People By Household Type[1]

	In Families			Unrelated Individuals		
Year	Total	Female Head[2]	Male Head[2]	Total	Female	Male
1960	87.6%	18.2	69.5	12.4	8.6	3.8
1965	85.5%	22.7	62.8	14.5	10.6	3.9
1970	80.0%	29.5	50.5	20.0	14.4	5.7
1975	80.3%	34.2	46.2	19.7	13.2	6.4
1980[3]	77.2%	34.6	42.6	21.3	14.1	7.2
1984[3]	78.5%	35.1	43.4	19.6	12.0	7.6

---

[1] Percentages may not add to 100 because of rounding.

[2] "Male head" and "Female head" are census terms. Male-headed households include married couple households and other households headed by a man.

[3] Includes unrelated subfamilies whose headship type cannot be identified from published data.

nearly five times as likely to be poor as men who head their own households. Unrelated women — who live alone or with others they are unrelated to — are somewhat more likely than unrelated men to be poor.

Over the past two-and-a-half decades the share of poor people living in female-headed households has doubled, rising from 18 to 35 percent. As Table 3 shows, by 1984 more than one in three poor people lived in a household headed by a woman, compared to half that many in 1959. These changes have been even more dramatic among blacks, where the percentage of poor in female-headed households has risen from 24.3 percent in 1959 to 59.7 percent in 1984. Among whites, 14.9 percent of the poor lived in female-headed households in 1959, and 25.6 percent in 1984.

By 1984, almost one in five poor people lived alone or in a household where they were unrelated to other individuals, and more than half of these poor were women. In contrast to the poor in female-headed households, however, the share of poor who are unrelated women is greater among whites than among blacks. The proportion of unrelated women has risen from 10.1 percent

Table 3
Poverty Rates of Various Groups of Women
and Men 15 Years Old and Older
-- 1984--

	Women	Men
Total[1]	14.1%	10.2%
Age		
15-17	17.9	18.0
18-21	19.0	15.7
22-24	17.7	13.5
25-34	14.4	9.4
35-44	11.5	8.0
45-54	10.7	8.0
55-59	11.1	8.6
60-64	12.6	8.9
65+	15.0	8.7
Race/Ethnicity[1],[2]		
White	11.5	8.4
Black	32.3	23.0
Hispanic	26.4	20.3
Marital Status[3]		
Single	19.9	15.1
Married, spouse present	7.7	7.7
Married, spouse absent	43.4	18.0
Widowed	23.4	17.8
Divorced	26.5	13.6
Household status[1]		
Spouse of head	6.9	6.9
Head of household	34.5	7.2
Unrelated	24.4	18.7

Source: Bureau of the Census, <u>Characteristics of the
Population Below the Poverty Level: 1984</u>. Current
Population Reports, Series P-60, No. 152.

---

[1] Data are for 1984.

[2] "White" and "Black" include Hispanics.

[3] Data on marital status are for 1983. In that year the
poverty rate for men 15 years old and over was 10.8 percent
and for women 15 years old and over 15.1 percent. Published
data for 1984 do not include tables for marital status.

of the white poverty population in 1959 to 14.2 percent in 1984,
compared to an increase from 4.9 to 7.2 percent over this same
time period among blacks.

There are as many poor married women as poor women who head households. Women who head their own households have the highest poverty rates of any group of household heads, and their share of the poverty population is growing rapidly. Nevertheless, there are as many poor married women as poor women who head their own households. And, as Table 4 shows, there are more poor unrelated women than either poor married women or poor female heads of households.

Thus the composition of a woman's household has a great deal to do with the likelihood that she will be poor and with the resources she can draw on to lift herself out of poverty. Closer examination of the characteristics of poor women in each household type unveils important differences within the population of poor women.

POOR MARRIED WOMEN

Published data on poor married women are not readily available, but their living situation can be surmised from analyses of statistics on male-headed households. More than 95 percent of the males who head households are married. As Figure 2 shows, the poverty rate for male-headed households follows a pattern similar to that for all people, but the rate of poverty is at a much lower level. The poverty rate for this group has hovered between 5 and 8 percent for the past two decades, in comparison to poverty rates between 11 and 17 percent for all people.

As the data in Table 5 show, however, the characteristics of poor male-headed households have changed over this time. Average household size has dropped and fertility has declined. Heads of poor households are younger, have more education, and are less likely to be full-time workers than household heads 25 years ago. Today's poor, married-couple household is less likely to be either a traditional "baby-boom" household where one wage-earner supports a large family or a retired couple. Rather, it is more likely that the poor married couple will be either a young household just starting out or a low-wage earning family in the prime of life.

More than two-thirds of poor male-headed households have at

Table 4

Characteristics of Poor Women 15 Years Old and Older
in 1984

	Percent of Poor Women	Number (1,000's)
Total[1]	100.0%	13,391
Age[1]		
15-17	7.2	961
18-21	11.1	1,485
22-24	8.4	1,120
25-34	22.3	2,987
35-44	13.8	1,842
45-54	9.2	1,234
55-59	5.0	663
60-64	5.4	729
65+	17.7	2,370
Race/Ethnicity[1],[2]		
White	70.1	9,384
Black	26.8	3,584
Hispanic	11.8	1,578
Marital Status[3]		
Single	30.3	4,298
Married, spouse present	27.5	3,909
Married, spouse absent	10.1	1,439
Widowed	18.2	2,588
Divorced	13.8	1,963
Household Status[1]		
Spouse of head	26.0	3,488
Head of household	26.1	3,498
Unrelated	30.1	4,035
Other family member	17.7	2,370

Source: Bureau of the Census, Characteristics of the
          Population Below the Poverty Level: 1984. Current
          Population Reports, Series P-60, No. 152

[1] Data are for 1984

[2] "White" and "Black" include Hispanics.

[3] Data on marital status are for 1983. In that year the
poverty rate for women 15 years old and over was 15.1 percent.
Published data for 1984 do not include tables for marital
status.

least one wage earner. In 1984, just over 70 percent of poor
male-headed families had at least one wage earner, and nearly
half of these families (31.9 percent of all poor male-headed

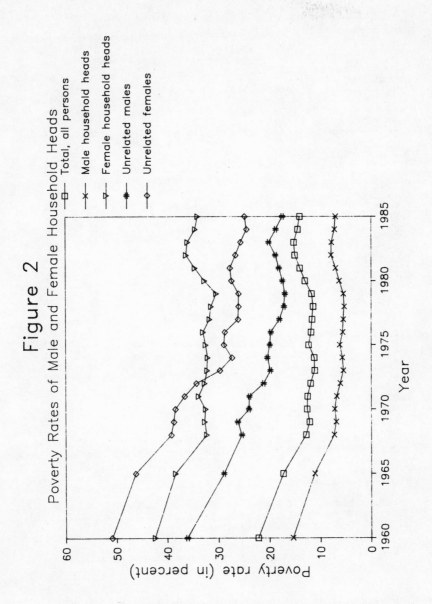

Figure 2

Poverty Rates of Male and Female Household Heads

— □ — Total, all persons
— × — Male household heads
— ▽ — Female household heads
— ✳ — Unrelated males
— ◇ — Unrelated females

Table 5

Characteristics of Poor Male-headed Households

	1984	1983	1980	1975	1970	1959
Age of Head						
15 to 24	9.6%	9.8%	9.7%	12.8%	9.1%	7.4%
25 to 44	47.5	48.3	43.6	36.2	32.0	37.6
45 to 54	14.9	13.3	14.4	15.0	13.0	16.8
55 to 65	14.7	14.3	12.4	16.7	16.3	14.3
65 and over	13.3	14.4	20.0	19.4	29.6	24.0
Average Family Size	3.64	3.88	3.85	3.95	3.88	4.30
Number of Children Under 18						
None	32.9	32.7	34.7	36.4	45.2	38.8
One	18.2	18.1	17.6	16.3	12.6	11.7
Two	22.0	22.0	20.0	15.1	11.6	13.5
Three or more	26.9	27.3	27.6	32.1	30.6	35.9
Educational Attainment of Household						
<High School	54.6	56.5	62.7	71.8	NA	NA
High school	28.7	28.6	24.2	17.1	NA	NA
Some college	16.7	14.9	13.1	11.1	NA	NA
Number of Workers[1]						
None	28.9	28.4	29.0	29.6	29.4	17.6
One	38.7	39.5	37.9	38.1	44.8	51.3
Two	25.4	25.4	25.1	23.7	19.2	22.3
Three or more	6.5	5.8	6.1	7.7	6.6	8.8
Labor Force Behavior of Head						
Worked	59.8	59.8	59.5	61.5	61.7	74.9
Year round/ full-time	26.1	26.2	25.6	24.2	27.9	37.6
Did not work	39.7	39.4	38.8	37.5	36.6	22.5

NA: Not available

Source: Bureau of the Census, Characteristics of the Population Below the Poverty Level: 1984. Current Population Reports, Series P-60, No. 152

---

[1] Published numbers do not total 100 percent.

households) had two or more workers in the household. This situation has remained relatively constant for the last 15 years.

Sixty percent of the men heading poor households worked in

1984. Over the past 15 years, roughly 60 percent of poor male-headed households have been headed by someone who worked at least part of the time during the year. As Table 5 shows, about a quarter of these households were headed by someone who worked year-round, full-time, which represents an approximate 10 percent decrease since 1959 in poor families whose head worked full-time, year-round.

The major reasons for the poverty male-headed households suffer is the lack of year-round, full-time work and the declining value of wages. During the 1960s and early 1970s, median earnings of full-time, year-round workers rose sharply; during the latter half of the 1970s median earnings were flat; and during the early 1980s they declined. This pattern is the inverse of the patterns of poverty in male-headed households, which suggests that their poverty rates are sensitive to economic conditions.

Nearly one in three poor male-headed households has two or more workers. In large part this increase in the number of workers is a result of the increased labor force participation rate of wives. As real wages declined, the labor-force participation of married women increased. By 1984, 40 percent of the wives in poor male-headed households worked, however, almost all of them worked part-time or part-year.

Men heading poor households have fewer resources to draw on for competing in the labor market than do men in general. More than half the heads of poor male-headed households (54.6 percent) dropped out of school before completing high school, compared to one in four men 18 years and older in the general population. Another 28.7 percent of poor male household heads have a high school degree only.

Male-headed households move in and out of poverty more quickly than other household types. Recent work by Bane and Ellwood (1986) shows that the major reason male-headed households enter poverty is loss of wages, and the major reason for leaving poverty is an increase in wages. In addition, the amount of time these households spend in poverty once entering it is less than that for almost every other type of household.

In 1984, fewer than one in five poor male-headed households received public assistance income. Poor male-headed households are more dependent on earnings than on public assistance for their well-being, with only 18.4 percent of male-headed households receiving any income from public assistance programs in 1984. Among younger households, the percentage was somewhat higher: one in four poor male-headed households with a head under 25 years received some public assistance during the year.

Low participation of poor male-headed households in public assistance programs is not surprising when current eligibility requirements are considered. Only about half the states have an Aid to Families with Dependent Children (AFDC) program for two-parent families with dependent children, and the general assistance programs for poor two-parent families tend to be small.

WOMEN HEADING THEIR OWN HOUSEHOLDS

Over the past several years a great deal of publicity has been given to the feminization of poverty, a term that refers to the rapid growth in the relative percentage of poor people living in female-headed households.

The share of poor people living in female-headed families has risen more rapidly than the share of the total population in this type of household. The growth in female-headed households is primarily attributable to the increasing divorce rate and decreasing marriage rate over the last three decades. In 1959, 8 percent of the population lived in female-headed households. By 1984, this percentage had risen to 13.2.

The increase in the poor living in female-headed families has been more rapid than its percentage increase in the general population. The percentage of the poor living in female-headed households has doubled since 1959, and now stands at 35 percent.

The poverty rate for female-headed households is much higher than that for any other household type. As Figure 2 shows, despite some gains made since 1959 in reducing their likelihood of being poor, by 1984 one in three women heading a household still had income below the poverty level. Among blacks and Hispanics, the rate was even higher: 52 and 53 percent, respectively.

Over the past 15 years, the number of elderly women heading poor households has declined. The proportion of poor female-headed households headed by elderly women dropped from 17 percent in 1959 to 6 percent in 1984. In part this decline is a reflection of the aging of the post-World War II baby boom generation. Children born during the baby boom years of 1945 to 1960 entered adulthood in the 1970s and 1980s in such large numbers that the share of all types of households headed by young adults increased dramatically.

The declining proportion of poor elderly women heading households also reflects the success of social programs in reducing poverty among the elderly. The proportion of elderly with income below the poverty level declined from 35 percent in 1959 to 12 percent in 1984. The greatest contributors to this decline have been entitlement programs such as Social Security, which has increased the scope of coverage and the real value of benefits over the past two decades, and Supplemental Security Income (SSI). Both of these programs are indexed, so their benefit levels keep pace with the rate of inflation.

Over the past 15 years, the average size of poor female-headed households has declined somewhat. As Table 6 shows, the average size of poor female-headed households dropped from 3.85 in 1970 to 3.39 in 1984. The small magnitude of this decline appears to result from two competing trends: an increase in the number of female-headed families with children, primarily reflective of the decreasing percentage of households headed by elderly women, and declining fertility. While more female-headed households today have children under age 18, there are fewer children in each.

More than one in three female household heads is in the labor force. In 1959 about 43 percent of female household heads held jobs and 15.8 percent worked year-round, full-time. By 1975 the percentage of female heads in the labor force had dropped to 36.5 percent, and has hovered at around that level ever since. The proportion of poor female household heads working year-round, full-time has fluctuated over the last 20 years, and was 12.6 percent of all poor women heading households in 1984.

Nearly half the poor female-headed households have at least one wage earner. In 1984, just under four in ten poor female-headed households had at least one person working, and 8.5 per-

Table 6

Characteristics of Poor Female-Headed Households

	1984	1983	1980	1975	1970	1959
Age of Householder						
15 to 24	15.9%	15.7%	17.0%	19.0%	14.5%	7.8%
25 to 44	59.8	58.9	59.0	56.5	50.9	47.4
45 to 54	11.1	11.3	10.8	11.8	15.4	18.9
55 to 65	7.1	7.3	6.9	6.7	8.5	9.0
65 and over	6.0	6.8	6.3	5.9	10.7	16.9
Average Family Size	3.38	3.39	3.41	3.64	3.85	3.66
Number of Children Under 18						
None	10.7%	12.4%	9.0%	7.3%	13.9%	20.4%
One	30.8	29.8	30.6	29.0	22.2	24.7
Two	29.8	29.2	30.5	25.1	21.8	19.4
Three or more	28.7	28.6	29.8	38.6	42.0	35.4
Educational Attainment of Householder						
∠high school	59.5	59.4	63.2	70.8	NA	NA
High School	27.8	29.8	27.2	23.7	NA	NA
Some college	12.7	10.8	9.6	5.5	NA	NA
Number of Workers						
None	52.6	53.9	50.8	52.7	45.2	44.6
One	38.9	37.6	39.6	37.8	41.5	38.8
Two	6.7	6.8	7.2	6.9	9.3	12.0
Three or more	1.8	1.7	2.4	2.6	4.0	4.6
Labor force behavior of head						
Worked	37.5	37.2	38.5	36.5	43.4	42.9
Year round/ full-time	12.6	10.9	10.1	9.2	12.1	15.8
Did not work	62.5	62.8	61.5	63.5	56.6	57.1

Source: Bureau of the Census, <u>Characteristics of the Population Below the Poverty Level: 1984</u>. Current Population Reports, Series P-60, No. 152.

cent had two or more members working. These percentages have remained relatively constant over the past 15 years.

Only four in ten poor women heading households have a high school degree. Six in ten poor women heading households dropped out of school before receiving a high school degree, in contrast to only one in four women over 18 in the general population. Thus, women heading poor households are at a disadvantage when it comes to competing in the labor market.

Only one in five poor women with children heading their own households receives any financial support from their children's fathers. Just over one in three poor women with children heading their own households in 1983 had a child support order, a legal agreement obligating the noncustodial parent to pay a given amount to the custodial parent toward the support of their children. Of this 35 percent with an order in place, one in three still received no money from the children's absent father. This represents only 13.5 percent of all poor women with children heading households. The remaining 64.5 percent of women with sole custodial care of their children had no child support order in place.

Nearly six in ten poor women heading households received public assistance in 1984. In 1984, 58 percent of all poor female-headed households received some income from public assistance. Among all poor households headed by women under age 25, 74.5 percent received income from public assistance.

TEENAGE MOTHERS: A SPECIAL CONCERN

Numerous studies have documented that women who begin parenting in their teens have fewer economic, social and emotional resources to draw on than do women who delay childbearing. Throughout their parenting years, early childbearers are much more likely to live in households with incomes below the poverty level. Among teen mothers, those who began parenting early are more likely to be poor at all ages than those who began parenting later in their teens.

Teenage fertility rates began dropping in the late 1950s. After 1960 fertility declined rapidly as women began delaying parenthood and spacing their children farther apart, an era demographers refer to as the "baby bust." Despite a general trend among all women, including teenagers, toward delaying childbearing, an increasing percentage of births in the 1960s and 1970s were to teens. This phenomenon reached its peak in 1973, when one out of every five children was born to a teenage mother. Among the black population one in three births was to a teen mother. The

explanation is that babyboomers born in the 1950s entered adolescence in the late 1960s and early 1970s in such large numbers
that a very large percentage of women of childbearing age were
teens.

The high poverty rates of women who began parenting in adolescence is attributable to three characteristics: fertility, labor
force participation on the part of mothers, and the probability of
having a spouse.

*Fertility rates have dropped faster for teenagers than for all
women over the last two decades. Nevertheless, teenagers still
have more children than their peers who delay childbearing.* The
poverty rate is a function of family size and income. Reducing
family size decreases the probability that a family will be poor,
all else remaining constant. Because teen mothers today have
fewer children, they have a greater chance of escaping poverty
than did teen mothers two decades ago. However, teen mothers
continue to have more children than their peers who delay parenting and teens who begin parenting in early adolescence have
more children than teens who begin parenting in late adolescence, a partial explanation of the higher poverty rates among
women who began parenting in adolescence.

*Teen mothers are less likely to ever marry than their peers who
delay fertility. Those teen mothers who do marry are more likely
than their peers to dissolve the relationship.* Demographic analyses suggest that although some unmarried teen mothers eventually marry, many do not. Three in ten teen mothers in 1980 had
not married: 16 percent of white teens and 72 percent of black
teens had not married. About 16 percent of women in their early
twenties in 1980 who had begun parenting in adolescence were
still unmarried.

Teen mothers also have higher divorce or separation rates than
their peers who delay parenting. Rates of marital disruption have
increased more rapidly for teen mothers over the past 20 years
than for women who delayed parenting.

Taken together, these trends suggest that teen mothers are less
likely than women who delay childbearing to have a spouse to
contribute to household earnings.

*The spouses of teen mothers who do marry tend to have lower
earnings than spouses of women who delay parenting.* Not only

do the spouses of teen mothers have lower earnings in young adulthood than the spouses of peers who delay parenting, but their earnings increase less rapidly as they age. This, combined with their average larger family size (greater fertility), makes it more difficult for the families of women who began parenting in adolescence to escape poverty.

Young teen mothers have lower rates of labor force participation than their peers who delayed parenting. Teen mothers are less dependent on their own earnings than women who delay parenting. About four in ten mothers between ages 15 and 19 were in the labor force in 1980. Fifty-five percent of the 20- to 24-year-old women who began parenting in their teens were in the labor force in 1980, in contrast to 62 percent of the 20- to 24-year-old mothers who delayed parenting until their early twenties.

Teen mothers are two to three times more likely to be receiving public assistance than their peers who delayed childbearing. Not only are women who begin parenting in their teens more likely than women who delay parenting to receive public assistance, once they begin to receive public assistance they tend to remain welfare clients longer. Recent research estimates that approximately 60 percent of the AFDC caseload is comprised of women who began parenting in adolescence.

Teen mothers are less educated than their peers who delay childbearing. Teen mothers are more likely to drop out of high school before graduation than their peers who delay parenting. The younger the teen mother, the more likely she is not to complete her education. Those who begin parenting before eighteen are much more likely than those who delay parenting until late adolescence to drop out of school early. Evidence suggests that early parenting does not stop a woman's educational attainment completely, but it does delay it. Over time, the educational attainment of teen mothers increases, but never reaches that of peers who delayed parenting.

Women who began parenting in adolescence would probably not be identical to their peers who delayed parenting if they too had waited to have their children. There are strong reasons to suspect that the gap between the two groups would be smaller if adolescents delayed fertility.

UNRELATED POOR WOMEN

Women who live alone, or are unrelated to other household members with whom they live, constitute an increased percentage of the poverty population over the past 25 years. Although the typical poor unrelated woman in 1984 was a 61-year-old who lived alone, there is a great diversity among this group. Approximately one in five poor unrelated women is under the age of 25. About 70 percent of this relatively young group is living in a household with other unrelated individuals, and nearly three-quarters are working. Fewer than 10 percent receive public assistance, SSI or any transfer payments.

However, half of poor unrelated women are elderly. More than two in five poor unrelated women are 65 or older; another 10 percent are aged 60 to 64. In contrast to their younger counterparts, nine in ten unrelated women over 65 live alone (see Table 7). Nine in ten receive Social Security payments; one in three receives Supplemental Security Income. Among blacks, half receive Supplemental Security Income. One in three poor elderly women receives some income from interest, dividends or rent. Among blacks the comparable share is one in six.

This suggests that among younger unrelated women poverty policies should center around labor market issues, and among the older group policies should center primarily around income-support programs. These strategies are presented more fully in the recommendations that follow.

POLICY PRESCRIPTIONS

The diversity among poor women suggests that there is no one strategy that will alleviate their poverty. Rather, we must consider multiple strategies, each of which addresses a subgroup of the population of poor women.

The most important antipoverty strategy we can pursue is creation of a productive, high-employment economy. As we have seen, many poor women work and most live in households where someone works. Their problem is low wages and too few hours. While this paper does not address macroeconomic issues, it is

Table 7

Age Distribution of Poor Household Heads
and Unrelated Individuals -- 1984

	Male Household Heads	Female Household Heads	Unrelated Males	Unrelated Females
15-17	*	*	1.9%	1.5%
18-21	3.8%	5.1%	13.0	10.7
22-24	5.7	10.6	14.3	6.7
25-34	26.4	36.5	22.5	9.3
35-44	21.1	23.2	11.6	5.1
45-54	14.9	11.1	9.2	7.7
55-59	7.3	3.8	6.4	6.6
60-64	7.4	3.3	5.4	9.7
65 and over	13.3	6.0	15.6	42.7
Average Age	41.6	34.3	34.2	61.2

* less than 0.5 percent

Source: Same as Table 6

clear that a society that tolerates a 7 percent unemployment rate will have poor people. And those with fewest resources to draw on — the poorly educated, single parents, disabled, and elderly — will have the greatest difficulty.

In addition to improving the economy, there are a range of policies that could be instituted to provide greater support to the poor who are currently working or who wish to be working. These include raising the minimum wage, providing health coverage to uninsured or inadequately insured working-poor families, and increasing the availability of and financial support for child care.

It is also clear that poor women and their spouses are less qualified than those with whom they compete for jobs. Improving the educational system, discouraging youth from dropping out of school and starting families too early, and extending opportunities to complete unfinished education and to upgrade skills in adulthood are essential anti-poverty strategies.

There is a need to increase the income support for poor women. Absent fathers must provide economic support to their children, rather than leaving mothers with full responsibility. Extending public assistance to two-parent families and increasing benefit levels to all eligible households would further diminish poverty.

It is clear from the data presented here that none of these strategies would be effective alone. Because of the great diversity of poor women, only a multifaceted antipoverty strategy will be effective.

REFERENCES

Bane, M. J. (1986). Household composition and poverty. In S. Danzinger and D. Weinberg, *Fighting Poverty: What Works and What Doesn't* (pp. 209-231). Cambridge, MA: Harvard University Press.

Bane, M. J. & Ellwood, D. (1986). Slipping into and out of poverty: The Dynamics of spells. *The Journal of Human Resources.* XXI, 1-23.

Moore, K. & Burt, M. (1982). *Private crisis, public cost: Policy perspective on teenage childbearing.* Washington, DC: Urban Institute Press.

U.S. Department of Commerce, Bureau of the Census (1985). *Characteristics of the population below the poverty level: 1983.* Current Population Reports, Series P-60. No. 147, Washington, DC: U.S. Government Printing Office.

U.S. Department of Commerce, Bureau of the Census (1986). *Characteristics of the population below the poverty level: 1984.* Current Population Reports, Series P-60, No. 152, Washington, DC: U.S. Government Printing Office.

U.S. Department of Commerce, Bureau of the Census (1986). *Child Support and Alimony: 1983.* Current Population Reports, Special Studies, Series P-23, No. 148, Washington, DC: U.S. Government Printing Office.

U.S. Department of Health, Education, and Welfare (1976). *The Measure of Poverty: A Report to Congress as Mandated by the Education Amendments of 1974.* Washington, DC: U.S. Government Printing Office.

Wilson, J. (1986). *Teenage parenting: The long-term effects for mothers and children.* Research Report R86-1 of the State, Local and Intergovernmental Center, John F. Kennedy School of Government, Harvard University. Cambridge, MA: John F. Kennedy School of Government.

The Health Plight
of Rural Women

Hila Richardson, DrPH

SUMMARY. All poor women have difficulty obtaining needed health services due to their poorer health status and lesser ability to pay for services. Rural poor women have additional conditions imposed on them by the isolation of the rural environment from resources commonly available in urban areas, such as public transportation to services and the availability of a wide range of health resources.

Strategies to address the health plight of rural women must first and foremost address their poverty. Strategies must also include a coherent national and state rural health policy that recognizes rural health as a distinct part of the larger health system.

INTRODUCTION

A woman trapped in poverty can have a despairing and tragic life no matter where she lives. However, the location of residence does determine the environment in which a woman must negotiate and manipulate her and her family's survival. The realities of life in both urban and rural areas determine the availability of resources and opportunities, and define the logistics necessary to find what is needed. This paper will discuss how the

Hila Richardson has a BS in Nursing from the University of Virginia and a Doctorate in Public Health from Columbia University. She is currently Associate Program Director of the Rural Hospital Program of Extended-Care Services, a national demonstration of The Robert Wood Johnson Foundation, administered by the Program in Health Policy and Management at New York University. She may be contacted through the Rural Hospital Program of Extended-Care Services, New York University, 113 University Place, New York, NY 10003.

The views expressed in this paper are solely those of Dr. Richardson and do not necessarily reflect the views of The Foundation or New York University.

41

realities of the rural environment determine rural women's health plight. After a brief general overview of rural women, including their health needs, the paper discusses the special problems faced by rural women in seeking health care in their communities and concludes by outlining a number of recommendations for the future.

RURAL WOMEN

Nearly 60 million people live in rural areas according to the 1980 census. Rural refers to the population living outside incorporated cities, villages, and boroughs of fewer than 2,500 inhabitants and it includes people living in rural parts of extended cities where there is low population density. Rural encompasses a wide range of lifestyles and levels of quality of life. Only 9.7 percent of the rural population is technically the farmer who conjures up images of rural life (U.S. Department of Commerce, 1983). In terms of the U.S. Census Bureau's two large categories that encompass the rural and urban areas, non-Metropolitan and Metropolitan Statistical Areas (MSAs), it is possible to live in a rural area inside an MSA. Or, a population may be technically non-MSA but live in a closely settled area with a central core that has a population of up to 50,000 residents — a "big city" to many rural people. About half, or 30 million, of the people living in rural areas are women. Although research focusing on rural women is just coming forth, a partial picture of their lives is emerging and, as in the general female population, age at marriage and divorce rates are increasing among rural women, while fertility and size of household are declining. In contrast to urban women, however, "rural women are still *more* likely to be married, have more children, live in larger families . . . complete their families earlier" but are less likely to divorce (Haney, 1982).

Occupational Status

Rural women are entering the paid work force in increasing numbers. During the 1960s and 1970s women accounted for nearly all the employment growth in nonmetropolitan counties. Particularly evident is the increased labor force participation of women with children. In a Michigan sample of farm families, except for large-scale farms, one-half or more of mothers with dependent children at home were employed off the farm (Haney, 1982).

Like urban women, rural women's jobs are concentrated in low-skill, low-wage occupations and industries. However, the differences in the types of industries (i.e., agriculture, textile, meat processing) in metropolitan and nonmetropolitan areas lead overall to an inferior economic situation for rural women. In addition, rural women have a more limited range of occupations, fewer chances for promotion, greater likelihood of part-time employment without benefits, including health insurance, and greater vulnerability to fluctuations in economic cycles (Haney, 1982). The lack of adult education, job-training programs, and child-care facilities in rural areas make it harder for women to overcome their inferior occupational status. Also, for the sizeable group of minority women in rural areas, the occupational problems are intensified by racism, language, and other cultural barriers to the jobs that are available. So, for example, in the South, black women are in the lowest paying and "dirtiest" jobs, while white women have the "cleaner" and relatively higher-paying clerical and front-office jobs (Smith, 1986).

Economic Status

A disproportionate number of rural women live in poverty, whether in intact families or in female-headed households. Table 1 shows that 37 percent of all U.S. families live in nonmetropolitan areas, both farm and nonfarm, but 40 percent of the families with incomes below $10,000 live in nonmetropolitan areas, with nonfarm populations having the highest proportion of poor families. One could argue that the cost of rent, food, and other necessities is higher in inner cities and, therefore, it is easier in a rural area to live on less than $10,000 a year. Although it is true the cost of living is higher in urban areas, it is also true that life in rural areas has hidden expenses. Because of the lack of public transportation, one of the largest expenses is buying and maintaining a personal car, a necessity for conducting simple daily tasks.

Table 1 also shows that a higher percentage of female-headed

TABLE 1

**All Families and Families with Female-Headed Households
By Residence and Income**

	Metropolitan			Non-Metropolitan	
	Total	Inner City	Outside Central City	Nonfarm	Farm
U.S. Families					
Number (in thousands)	61,019	15,838	27,774	19,104	1,303
Percent	100	26	41	31	6
U.S. Families with incomes below $10,000					
Number (in thousands)	10,552	3,386	2,917	3,882	367
Percent	100	32	28	37	3
U.S. Female Households[1]					
Number (in thousands)	9,404	3,607	3,226	2,513	58
Percent of all Families	15	23	12	13	4
Female Households with income below $10,000					
Number (in thousands)	4,309	1,136	1,864	1,278	31
Percent	48	59	31	51	53

[1] Without husband present

Source: U.S. Bureau of the Census (1981). Current Population Reports: Money, Income of Household, Families and Persons in U.S. Table 21. Washington: D.C. U.S. Government Printing Office.

households in both farm and nonfarm rural areas have low incomes. Although 17 percent of rural families are headed by females, more than half of those families have a total income of less than $10,000 a year. In addition to low occupational status, another contributing factor to this impoverishment are the more limited benefits of public assistance programs in rural areas. Both the conservative nature of local governments and the small tax base of rural communities lead to lower per capita expenditures for services provided by local governments (Rogers, 1982).

Rural poverty usually has been associated with the Southeast, the Appalachia area, and some parts of the Southwest. The recent crisis in the farm economy and the subsequent loss of more than a million jobs on farms and other rural businesses in the Midwest and in North Central states, however, have created areas of rural poverty in the "farm belt" (Schneider, 1986). Counties where people have trouble purchasing food or qualifying for food stamps have shifted, from the South to the Southwest to the bread-belt states of Iowa, Missouri, North Dakota, South Dakota, Nebraska, and Montana. The Nebraska Division of Family Services reports that food stamp applications increased almost 25 percent between 1983 and 1985 (Physicians Task Force on Hunger in America, 1986).

THE HEALTH PLIGHT OF POOR RURAL WOMEN

The basis of rural women's health plight is their poverty, which is associated with poorer health status and lesser ability to pay for services. While poverty imposes these conditions on all poor women, the rural environment imposes the additional conditions of lack of transportation and fewer available resources.

Health Status

Data on the health status of all rural women are almost nonexistent and even more scarce for poor, rural women. Information must be extrapolated largely from data on general rural and poverty populations. The health status of the general rural population compares favorably with the urban population with respect to death rates and the incidence of acute conditions (U.S. Department of Health and Human Services, 1984). Residents in rural areas, however, have higher rates of many chronic conditions, with the greatest differences in incidences of arthritis, back disorders, bursitis, hearing and visual impairments, ulcers, and hernias.

Chronic conditions restrict activity to a greater degree for rural than urban residents. A higher percentage of rural persons with chronic conditions are limited or unable to carry out their major activities (U.S. Department of Health and Human Services, 1984). A number of these conditions are related to the dangers of working outside and with the heavy machinery associated with farming, logging, mining, and millwork. Although women are seldom employed in such heavier industrial work they do farm and work in jobs with special occupational risks, such as operatives in textile and apparel manufacturing and poultry and meat processing (see Stellman, this volume).

Health risks increase as income decreases. The effects of a lifestyle that includes poor nutrition, inadequate housing, and unsafe living and working environments are realized in lower life expectancy, higher mortality, particularly infant and maternal mortality, and more chronic diseases, especially for blacks and other minorities (U.S. Department of Health and Human Services, 1980; 1985).

Socioeconomic conditions, stress, and emotional and behavioral functioning are positively correlated and rural women share many of the same stressful life events as urban women. Rural women, however, report more stress related to environmental-related events, such as severe weather, natural disasters, changes in nature, size of community, and economic conditions (Bigbee, 1985). Recent reports of suicides and homicides in economically depressed farm communities have focused attention on the severe effects of stress and depression on families. A survey of farm families conducted by Iowa State University found that 20 percent reported experiencing a great deal of stress on a day-to-day basis; 42 percent acknowledged having stress; and 18 percent were very concerned about their level of stress (Northwest Health Services, Inc. et al., 1986). When primary-care physicians were surveyed, 62 percent reported they had observed an increase in stress-related problems since 1983.

Less Ability to Pay

Although financial barriers to health services are not unique to poor rural women, the proportion of low-income people without any type of health insurance, public or private, is higher in nonmetropolitan areas. In 1984, 34.2 percent of the uninsured below the poverty level lived in nonmetropolitan areas compared to

33.2 percent who lived in inner cities. In the general rural population, 20 percent are uninsured compared to 15.2 percent of the general U.S. population (Sulvetta & Swartz, 1986).

The main obstacle to private health insurance coverage for rural residents is the limited availability of employee plans through small retail operations, locally owned mills, and self-employed farmers, which generally offer little or no health insurance coverage. A woman in a low-paying job ($400-$700 per month) who buys her own health insurance in North Carolina might have to pay $80 to $130 monthly for herself and her children. One can expect an additional $1,000 in uninsured deductibles annually (Arnold, 1986). Individual policies also may have restricted coverage for certain conditions or lower limits on payments for various procedures. One large employer in the Southeast, which does provide health insurance to its 4,000 employees, largely women with children, includes $100 limits on hospital rooms, physician visits, and prescription drugs. Surgical procedures are covered at about one-fourth the actual cost, and payment for a normal childbirth is limited to $200 when the usual fee in the area is at least $1,000 (Arnold, 1986).

At a recent hearing on the uninsured in rural Wisconsin, a woman from a family of four with an income of $8,000 annually and a $1,000 deductible on her husband's employee health insurance stated:

> The health insurance we have is paid through my husband's employer but it hardly covers anything unless it is large or major. . . . Because we end up paying all of our bills anyway, it is like we have no insurance at all. It is very discouraging when we pay each month and get no benefit from it. (Drake & Peterson, 1985)

With a disproportionate percentage of the poor and uninsured, rural areas should logically equal or exceed urban areas in the use of federal Medicaid and Medicare programs aimed at these populations. However, these federal programs discriminate against rural areas. The major problem with Medicaid is that it is tied to state welfare eligibility criteria and in rural states of the West, Northwest, North Central, and South, such eligibility is likely to be limited to aged poor, disabled, and single-parent families.

Fewer than 20 percent of the families with incomes below
$10,000 in farm and nonfarm rural areas are headed by a female
and qualify as a single-parent family, in contrast to almost 30
percent of families in urban areas.

Rural states also have lower income eligibility standards for
welfare. Nationwide, the average monthly Medicaid eligibility
level was $319 per month for a family of four in 1985, or 38
percent of the federal poverty income level of $850 per month. In
thirteen of seventeen rural states in the South Atlantic, East
South Central, and West South Central, the eligibility level for
Medicaid fell below this national average. In Alabama and
Texas, monthly income eligibility for Medicaid is 17 percent and
21 percent of the federal poverty level, respectively (National
Health Law Program, 1985).

Medicare is also biased against rural areas in that coverage is
limited to those who qualify for Social Security or for railroad
retirement benefits. Self-employed farmers and their wives, mi-
grant workers, part-time workers, all of whom are concentrated
in rural areas, usually do not pay regularly into Social Security
and, therefore, are not eligible for Medicare coverage when they
turn 65 years of age. (Medicare hospitalization and physician
premiums can be purchased but the annual premium is more than
$1,000.)

Medicare also pays rural physicians lower rates, averaging
about 75 percent of those in metropolitan counties (Walleck &
Kretz, 1981). Lower fees with the same complicated billing system discourages physicians from accepting Medicare patients or
encourages them to charge additional fees. Elderly women may
not benefit at all from Medicare if they are not eligible for Social
Security or if their local physician does not accept Medicare.
Their only recourse is to pay out-of-pocket or attempt to qualify
for Medicaid.

Lack of Transportation

Lack of public transportation in rural areas creates a particularly difficult barrier to care for poor women. A private car is
often the only option available for traveling to health services.
Yet, in a survey of low-income rural communities, only 20 per-

cent of the population owned their own car (Kaye, 1982). Without public transportation, poor women must depend on the willingness of neighbors or family to take them to physicians or to hospital care. The sense of helplessness this situation causes is clear from the tragic example described by a woman in a rural area of North Carolina:

> We recognize the presence of physicians who are within a 3-10 mile radius, and a local physician who does not accept Medicaid, Medicare or insurance. Give these statistics to Mrs. Jones, whose child is lying on the bed, not moving, not breathing, she does not own a car, has no money and no one to take her to the doctor's office. She calls the doctor, tells him her child's condition and the doctor says, "your child is dead." (Fremont Concerned Citizens, 1986)

Fewer Services Available

For both the poor and nonpoor in rural areas, there are fewer health services available. Although the federal programs of the 1960s and 1970s stimulated growth in health-related services to rural areas, there remains a wide gap in the availability of health resources, particularly for health personnel (Rosenblatt & Moscovice, 1982). In 1986, two-thirds of the 1,906 areas designated by the federal government as shortage areas for primary-care physicians, dentists, and psychiatrists were in nonmetropolitan areas. Of the 34.5 million people living in a designated shortage area, 16.2 million, nearly half, lived in nonmetropolitan shortage areas (U.S. Department of Health and Human Services, 1986). Almost 30 percent of the rural population lives in an area with a shortage of primary care providers, despite the nationwide surplus of physicians and their recent shift to areas outside urban centers (Schwartz et al., 1986).

The shortage of board-certified specialists is even greater. There were 2.5 and 2.4 obstetricians/gynecologists (OB/GYNs) and pediatricians, respectively, per 100,000 persons in nonmetropolitan areas in contrast to 7.7 OB/GYNs and 9.1 pediatricians per 100,000 persons in 1977 in metropolitan areas (Schwartz et al., 1980). A family practitioner can provide the basic OB/GYN or pediatric services. Less than half the communities with a population of 2,500 to 5,000, however, had a family practitioner in 1977 and only about two-thirds of the communities with 5,000 to 10,000 people had family practitioners (Schwartz et al., 1980).

Another factor that may contribute to an increase in the physician shortage in rural areas is the current economic crisis on farms. Primary-care physicians surveyed in Iowa, Missouri, Kansas, and Nebraska reported that since 1981 they had experienced a decrease in utilization, an increase in accounts receivable, and an increase in patients who cannot pay (Northwest Health Services, Inc. et al., 1986). This economic situation may force physicians to leave for a larger population base.

Other shortages of personnel include registered nurses and specialists in ancillary areas such as physical therapy, respiratory therapy, radiology, and laboratory services. It is difficult to recruit new personnel to remote rural areas. Hospitals and clinics that require these specialties may have to offer salaries competitive with urban areas. Even when recruitment is successful, there is frequent turnover due to difficulties in adjusting to rural life.

In addition to personnel shortages, many rural areas lack access to hospital beds. Although there are about 2,900 rural hospitals in the U.S., they are not always distributed according to need. Approximately two-thirds have fewer than 100 beds, tend to be older, less well-equipped and less likely to have specialized personnel such as X-ray technicians and physical therapists. The increasingly competitive health-care environment, changes in payment for Medicare beneficiaries, and loss of patients to larger hospitals in cities also threaten rural hospitals (American Hospital Association, 1985).

At the same time, the rural hospital is an important community resource. It is often the first or second largest area employer and purchaser and is central to attracting and keeping physicians. As a result, rural communities show strong support for the hospitals and have even increased local taxes to make up for the loss of other hospital revenue (American Hospital Association, 1985).

Emergency services are another area of urban and rural difference. Emergency services are seldom available in rural areas, largely because it is not economically feasible to support a full-time emergency team in sparsely populated areas. The emergency services that do exist are usually hospital-based and often staffed by volunteers with varying degrees of training and experience. In addition, volunteer response time is longer, causing more loss of life during the wait for ambulances (Rosenblatt & Moscovice, 1982). In rural hospitals that do provide professionally staffed emergency services, a nurse on duty "floats" to the emergency room as needed. If necessary, she will then contact a physician, who may or may not be in the hospital at the time.

The combination of less available services and large expanses of land in rural areas make rural people more likely to travel longer distances often over dangerous road conditions. A national survey comparing travel times in 1976 found that 12 percent of the rural population traveled more than 30 minutes to health services, the accepted maximum, while only 6 percent of the urban population traveled that long (Aday et al., 1980). The direct and indirect costs of extended travel time to health services discourage the use of those services.

Utilization of Services

Rural residents see physicians less often each year than do urban residents, with 4.5 physician contacts each year compared to 5.3 for those in urban areas (U.S. Department of Health and Human Services, 1984). Data comparing the proportions of some acute conditions that receive medical attention in the SMSA and non-SMSA populations show that for most conditions the rural and urban utilization patterns are about the same. These acute conditions are generally more difficult to cure without treatment and medications, and include urinary-track infections, fractures and dislocations, open wounds and lacerations, and acute bronchitis. Problems that require some minimal primary medical care, such as infectious and parasitic diseases, chronic childhood diseases, acute ear infections, disorders of menstruation, and acute musculoskeletal conditions, received less attention in rural areas. Rural residents may let these conditions "run their course" and not consider it worth the time and money to see a physician (U.S. Department of Health and Human Services, 1984).

Hospital discharge rates (excluding childbirth) are 13.2 per

100 persons in rural areas and 11 per 100 persons for urban residents (U.S. Department of Health and Human Services, 1984). This difference might be explained partly by the unavailability of physicians and health insurance, causing rural residents to postpone care until longer hospitalization is required. Another possible explanation may be differences in physician-admitting practices when patients must travel long distances for daily treatments that could be provided on an outpatient basis in an urban area.

SUMMARY AND RECOMMENDATIONS

The health plight of rural women is rooted in poverty, which contributes to their poorer health status and creates financial barriers to obtaining health care. The rural environment adds another dimension to this plight brought on by more difficult access to private or public health insurance and to transportation services. And in comparison to urban areas, there are fewer services available in rural communities.

The special needs of rural women can be addressed through policies that diminish poverty and provide protection through a national health program for uninsured populations. In addition, there must be initiatives on the national, state, and local levels that recognize rural health services as a distinct part of the total health system. The problems of rural health cannot be solved by piecemeal tinkering with the health policies and regulations directed at urban providers. Rural health policies and programs must specifically target the shortages of personnel and resources and the lack of transportation, in addition to inadequate insurance.

National and state-level agencies designated for the purpose of defining the rural health problems and developing coherent strategies and policies to address these issues are needed. Some other strategies could include:

To improve health insurance coverage:

— eliminating Medicaid eligibility criteria tied to state welfare eligibility.

— developing incentives for small businesses to provide adequate health insurance coverage for employees.
— restructuring or supplementing Medicaid and Medicare to cover self-employed farmers, seasonal workers, and others who fall between the cracks of eligibility requirements.

To increase availability of services:

— reimbursing physicians and hospitals such that the costs associated with recruiting personnel to remote areas and serving a low volume of patients are recognized.
— establishing or reinstituting federal and state programs that encourage health personnel through educational loans or tax incentives to practice in rural areas.

To improve transportation:

— setting up special loan programs for rural providers or communities to upgrade facilities and to provide transportation services.

On a local level, rural communities and providers should plan jointly for improved use of existing resources and develop strategies for attracting new resources. Also, community businesses and civic organizations should develop resources and means to provide transportation services. Although these changes are not specifically directed at poor rural women, they would increase the resources available in the rural health environment in which she must function. Ultimately, however, her underlying plight of poverty must be specifically addressed through changes in social and economic policies.

REFERENCES

Aday, L. A., Andersen, R. & Fleming, G. V. (1980). *Health care in the U.S.* Beverly Hills: Sage Publications, Inc.

American Hospital Association (1985). Rural hospitals face upheaval. *Media background sheet.* Chicago: American Hospital Association, No. 8.

Arnold, C. (1986). *Testimony to North Carolina Indigent Health Care Study Commission.* Murfreesboro, NC: Center for Women's Economic Alternatives.

Bigbee, J. L. (1985). Stressful life events among women: A rural-urban comparison. Doctoral Dissertation. University of Wyoming, School of Nursing.

Drake, J. & Peterson, R. (1985). *The needs of Wisconsin's rural uninsured.* Madison, WI: Center for Public Representation.

Fremont Concerned Citizens (1986). Testimony to North Carolina Indigent Health Care Study Commission. Fremont, North Carolina.

Haney, W. G. (1982). Women. In D. A. Dillman & D. J. Hobbs (Eds.), *Rural society in the U.S.* Boulder: Westview Press.

National Health Law Program (1985). New state statistics on percentage of poor covered by Medicaid. *Health Advocate.* Los Angeles: National Health Law Program.

Northwest Health Services, Inc. and Midwest Rural Health Association (1986). *Rural health crisis.* Mound City and Kansas City, MO.

Physician Task Force on Hunger in America (1986). *Hunger counties 1986: The distribution of America's high-risk areas.* Boston: Harvard University School of Public Health.

Rogers, D. L. (1982). Community services. In D. A. Dillman & D. J. Hobbs (Eds.), *Rural society in the U.S.* Boulder: Westview Press.

Rosenblatt, R. A. & Moscovice, I. S. (1982). *Rural health care.* New York: John Wiley & Sons.

Schneider, K. (1986). Upheaval in U.S. food industry forces a hard look at its future. *New York Times.* October 9, 1986.

Schwartz, W. B., Newhouse, J. P., Bennett, B. W. & Williams, A. P. (1980). *The changing geographic distribution of board-certified physicians.* Los Angeles: The Rand Corporation.

Smith, B. E. (1986). North Carolina: Who benefits from "economic" development. *Voices of the rural south.* Lexington, KY: Southeast Women's Employment Coalition.

Stellman, J. M. (1987). The working environment of the working poor: An analysis based on workers' compensation claims, census data and known risk factors. *Women and Health* (this issue).

Sulvetta, M. B. & Swartz, K. (1986). *The uninsured and uncompensated care.* Washington, DC: National Health Policy Forum, George Washington University.

U.S. Bureau of the Census (1983). *General social and economic characteristics.* Washington, DC: U.S. Government Printing Office.

U.S. Department of Health and Human Services, Bureau of Health Professions, Office of Data Analysis (1986). *Selected statistics on health manpower shortage areas.* Monograph.

_____ (1984). *Current estimate for the National Health Interview Survey.* Series 10, No. 156. Washington, DC: U.S. Government Printing Office.

_____ Public Health Service, Health Resources Administration, Office of Resources Opportunity (1980). *Health of the disadvantaged.* Washington, DC: U.S. Government Printing Office.

_____ (1985). *Report of the secretary's task force on black and minority health.* Washington, DC: U.S. Government Printing Office.

Walleck, S. S. & Kretz, S. E. (1981). *Rural Medicine.* Lexington, MA: D.C. Heath & Company.

Women and Poverty:
The Effects on Reproductive Status

Lorna McBarnette, MS, MPH

SUMMARY. National surveys, over the years, have provided evidence of relationship between poverty and health. In the United States, access to health care is generally dependent on the ability to pay for it. As a consequence, poor women are dependent upon government-funded social-welfare programs to attain access to health care. This paper examines the relationship between poverty and several indicators of reproductive status, and concludes that there is a relationship between poverty and poor reproductive status. The health gap between poor and nonpoor women is related to the absence of financial and other resources that dictate lifestyle.

INTRODUCTION

The term "the feminization of poverty" which was introduced by Pearce and McAdoo (1981) very aptly makes a connection between women and poverty that is indicative of the social and economic conditions that affect women as a group. This connection between women and poverty is real. Women and children are the primary beneficiaries of social-welfare programs for the poor. Between the mid-1960s and the mid-1970s, the number of poor adult males declined, while the number of the poor in households headed by women increased by 100,000 a year. By

Lorna McBarnette is Executive Deputy Commissioner, New York State Department of Health, Corning Tower, 14th Floor, Albany, NY 12237. The following Department staff provided assistance: M. Gesche, MD, MPH, MA, Bureau of Reproductive Health; V. Logrillo, MPH and G. Therriault, MSPH, Bureau of Biostatistics; P. Nasca, PhD and A. Weinstein, MPH, Bureau of Cancer Epidemiology; D. Murphy, Bureau of Communicable Disease; M. E. Henry, AIDS Institute.

55

1980, the poor in the United States were predominantly female; two out of three adults who fell below the official federal poverty line were women, and more than half of the families who were poor were headed by women (Ehrenreich & Piven, 1985). In 1983, 35 percent of all poor people lived in families headed by women, as compared to 17.8 percent in 1959 (O'Hare, 1985); nearly half of the nation's 7.2 million families in 1985 were headed by women (Wall Street Journal, 8/27/86); and, the most significant characteristic of female-headed households is their poverty (Moore & Burt, 1982).

National surveys over the years have provided evidence of yet another connection—between poverty and ill health—as evidenced by the poorer health status of low-income people. Sixty percent of children coming from families defined as poor have one or more chronic diseases (White, 1968). The incidence of all forms of cancer is inversely related to income (Dorn & Cutler, 1951). Heart disease and diabetes are more prevalent among the poor (Ellis, 1958). Infant mortality rises considerably as income decreases; and for the poor, the risk of dying under the age of 25 is four times the national average (US DHEW, 1973).

Unfortunately, many professionals working in the field of health do not view poverty as a health problem. They view the poverty syndrome, which leads to chronic low socioeconomic status, as something outside the boundaries of health, requiring corrective actions that are unrelated to the goals of the health care system. Fortunately, there are others who believe that an appreciation of the relationship between poverty and ill health can serve as a trigger mechanism that could possibly lead to development and implementation of social and health policies that offer solutions to both poverty and poor health status (Newell, 1984).

Within the narrower framework of women, poverty, and reproductive status there is evidence that poverty is a constraint in terms of access to health and medical services during and after reproductive events; and although strides have been made in rectifying the disparity between poor and nonpoor women, economic deprivation is still associated with poorer health, and the quantity and quality of health and medical services received by the poor is below the national average (Kane, Kasteler & Gray, 1976). Poverty in the United States has always been disproportionately concentrated among minorities. In recent years, however, with the increasing number of women who are poor, there has occurred a convergence between class and gender that is unprecedented in American history (Ehrenreich & Piven, 1985).

ACCESS TO HEALTH SERVICES

The reliance of women on social-welfare programs for some measure of economic security has risen in concert with the increase in poverty among women. In the United States, access to health care is generally dependent on the ability to pay for it. As a consequence, poor women are dependent on government-funded social-welfare programs to attain access to health services. In 1980, Medicaid covered only 39.1 percent of the population below the poverty level and 4.0 percent of the population above the poverty level. Of the white poor, only 39.9 percent were covered, compared to 65.1 percent of the black poor, and 46.6 percent of Hispanics. Of the near-poor (101-150 percent of poverty), 14.7 percent of whites, 25.1 percent of blacks, and 28.8 percent of Hispanics had Medicaid coverage in 1980 (US DHHS, 1985).

The number of obstetricians and gynecologists who provide specialized reproductive care, and participate in the Medicaid program, or treat uninsured women is decreasing. In 1985, four out of ten physicians who provided obstetrical services did not accept Medicaid clients both for payment and liability reasons, according to a report released by the Alan Guttmacher Institute (1985). The study concluded that the health of mothers appears to be suffering in large part because of compromised access to prenatal care. In 1982, 42 percent of all births involved women ages 18-24, but more than one in four of those women had neither public nor private health insurance (Guttmacher Institute, 1985). In New York State, the Medicaid maximum allowable fee is such that, in the marketplace, specialist care for poor women is almost unavailable (US DHHS, Report of the Secretary's Task Force on Black and Minority Health, 1986). National data suggest obstetricians and gynecologists, in fact, have lower than average Medicaid participation rates than all other primary care physicians, and they are less likely to accept Medicaid patients than the majority of secondary specialists (Center for Health Economics Research, 1982).

A higher proportion of poor women consistently receives inadequate prenatal care. The experience in New York State, for example, is instructive in terms of the differentials between poor and nonpoor women, and between women residing in urban and rural or suburban areas. In New York City, the percentage of women with inadequate prenatal care is consistently higher than in Upstate New York, regardless of poverty status or race. The overall risk of having inadequate prenatal care is nearly 150 percent higher for poor women in New York City (see Table 1) than for women with private insurance, and is 74 percent higher for poor women in Upstate New York (see Table 2). Poor women are also more likely to have a low birthweight infant. The excess risk in New York City is estimated at 46 percent (see Table 3), compared to 20 percent in Upstate New York (see Table 4) (New York State Department of Health, Bureau of Biostatistics, 1986).[1]

Many low-income women have part-time or low-paying jobs that do not provide health insurance benefits. In 1984, women were disproportionately represented among New Yorkers working part-time, but indicating a preference for full-time work, 56.6 percent, as compared to their representation among the total employed, 43.4 percent (New York State Department of Labor, 1986). There are approximately 44,000 women residing in identified "high risk" areas of New York State who become pregnant, are not eligible for Medicaid, and who do not have other forms of health insurance (New York State Department of Health, Bureau of Reproductive Health, 1985).

POVERTY AND REPRODUCTIVE TRENDS

The women's liberation movement and the almost concurrent advent of the very effective female methods of contraception such as the "pill" freed women, including the very young, from dependence on the male for protection against pregnancy. During the last two decades, these phenomena together have had a profound effect on both the style and outcomes of women's repro-

TABLE 1
PERCENTAGE WITH INADEQUATE PRENATAL CARE *
BY RACE AND HEALTH INSURANCE STATUS
NEW YORK CITY   RECORDED 1985

NON HISPANIC WHITES		TOTAL
MEDICAID	1,019 (31.5%)	3,236
THIRD PARTY INSURANCE	1,804 (6.2%)	29,277

NON HISPANIC BLACKS		
MEDICAID	5,732 (37.5%)	15,288
THIRD PARTY INSURANCE	2,243 (17.5%)	12,832

HISPANIC		
MEDICAID	5,403 (33.0%)	16,352
THIRD PARTY INSURANCE	2,139 (21.2%)	10,040

* AS DEFINED BY THE KESSNER INDEX (REFERENCE ATTACHED).

ductive behavior, and indirectly on the relationship between women and poverty.

The period of adolescence is a difficult time for girls because of the extended time period between physical sexual maturity and emotional, societal and economic maturity. In addition, the tendency toward risk-taking behavior in the young, coupled with peer pressure, militate against young girls, on their own, refraining from initiating early sexual activity. And, despite the increased acceptance of "women's lifestyles," there continues to be a double standard for acceptable behavior.

Among women under 20 years of age, the proportion at risk of unintended pregnancy is lower for those in higher-income fam-

ilies (Torres, 1983) and young women with higher educational
expectations are less likely to initiate sex at an early age. The
same holds for the young from intact families (Moore & Burt,
1982). Educated women, by virtue of their education, have already escaped the probability of becoming poor. However, all
young women, particularly before they complete their education,
are at risk of early unintended pregnancy.

Early child-bearing is strongly associated with decreased educational attainment, and young mothers, very seldom "catch
up" educationally with their counterparts who postponed childbearing (Moore & Waite, 1977; Mott & Marsiglio, 1985). And,
low educational attainment is strongly associated with subse-

TABLE 2
PERCENTAGE WITH INADEQUATE PRENATAL CARE *
BY RACE AND SOCIO-ECONOMIC STATUS
UPSTATE NEW YORK RESIDENTS 1985

NON HISPANIC WHITES		TOTAL
LOW SES AREAS	902 (10.8%)	8,320
OTHER SES AREAS	6,897 (6.0%)	114,023
NON HISPANIC BLACKS		
LOW SES AREAS	1,075 (24.3%)	4,424
OTHER SES AREAS	1,365 (16.7%)	8,153
HISPANIC		
LOW SES AREAS	159 (17.9%)	890
OTHER SES AREAS	493 (11.9%)	4,129

* AS DEFINED BY THE KESSNER INDEX (REFERENCE ATTACHED).

TABLE 3
PERCENTAGE OF LIVE BIRTHS WITH
BIRTHWEIGHT UNDER 2500 GRAMS
BY RACE AND HEALTH INSURANCE STATUS
NEW YORK CITY   RECORDED 1985

NON HISPANIC WHITES		TOTAL
MEDICAID	207 (6.4%)	3,236
THIRD PARTY INSURANCE	1,165 (4.0%)	29,277

NON HISPANIC BLACKS		
MEDICAID	1,906 (12.5%)	15,288
THIRD PARTY INSURANCE	1,119 (8.7%)	12,832

HISPANIC		
MEDICAID	1,226 (7.5%)	16,352
THIRD PARTY INSURANCE	567 (5.6%)	10,040

quent poverty. As a consequence of fewer and less marketable skills and limited employment opportunities, a large percentage of these young women end up on public assistance, that is, they become poor, and very often, they remain poor. Mothers without a high school education are nearly twice as likely to live in households receiving Aid to Families with Dependent Children (AFDC) as compared to women with a high school education (Moore & Burt, 1982). And, according to Reid (1982), the larger proportion of poor families among blacks when compared with whites is correlated to their higher overall fertility.

Birth rates for unmarried women ages 15-19 have risen almost uninterrupted from 1940 through 1980, due primarily to the lesser inclination of adolescent women to legitimize births before marriage; and, women who begin childbearing in their teens tend to have more births subsequently than women who delay child-bearing until their twenties (Thorton & Freedman, 1983). Black women are more likely to bear a child as a teenager and to have an unplanned birth, although the incidence of out-of-wedlock births in white teenagers has increased more than in any other ethnic group of the same age. An analysis from the National Survey of Family Growth (NSFG) found that the probability of a pregnancy during the first year following a first birth for all teen mothers was 17 percent, with the pregnancy rates among women with incomes less than 150 percent of poverty twice as high as

TABLE 4
PERCENTAGE OF LIVE BIRTHS WITH
BIRTHWEIGHT UNDER 2500 GRAMS BY
RACE AND SOCIO-ECONOMIC STATUS
UPSTATE NEW YORK RESIDENTS 1985

NON HISPANIC WHITES		TOTAL
LOW SES AREAS	545 (6.5%)	8,349
OTHER SES AREAS	5,759 (5.0%)	114,547

NON HISPANIC BLACKS		
LOW SES AREAS	562 (12.6%)	4,452
OTHER SES AREAS	1,011 (12.3%)	8,191

HISPANIC		
LOW SES AREAS	75 (8.3%)	901
OTHER SES AREAS	243 (5.9%)	4,135

those in women with higher income (Ford, 1983). Demographically, the increase in female-headed families since 1960 is linked to the rising proportion of children born out of wedlock and the increase in divorce, although the divorce rate has levelled off since 1981 (O'Hare, 1985).

The New York State experience shows that for both New York City and Upstate women, there is a clear difference in the level of out-of-wedlock births between the poor and the nonpoor. For third-party (other than Medicaid) funded births, the proportions that occurred among married non-Hispanic whites, non-Hispanic blacks and Hispanics were 95 percent, 61 percent, 74 percent respectively. For the Medicaid-supported births, the proportion of married women among the three groups was much smaller, namely 57 percent, 17 percent, and 35 percent respectively (see Table 5). Births that occur to poor women in New York City are nearly seven times as likely to be out of wedlock as in wedlock. In Upstate New York, poor women are two and one-half times more likely to be unwed at the time of delivery (see Table 6) (New York State Department of Health, Bureau of Biostatistics, 1986).

An Urban Institute study found that when welfare dependency is used to measure persistent poverty, fewer than 10 percent of mothers receiving AFDC payments stayed on welfare for ten consecutive years (O'Hare, 1985). Nevertheless, teenage mothers are disproportionately recipients of public assistance. As reported by Moore and Burt (1982), of recipients under the age of 30, the majority were teenagers at first childbirth; 64 percent in 1975 and 1977, according to Scheirer; 71 percent in 1975 according to Moore, et al.; and, 80 percent in Monroe County, New York during 1977 and 1978 as calculated by Block.

Moore and Burt (1982) hypothesize that "teens, especially poor and minority teens, may perceive less incentive to avoid early child bearing because discrimination limits their future opportunities." A variety of reasons is indicated for this. One holds that perhaps young women have a disincentive to do so, in as much as the welfare system is structured so that marriage precludes eligibility for AFDC. There is no evidence to indicate that public-welfare assistance serves as an economic incentive for early sexual activity or pregnancy. As most of these pregnancies

TABLE 5
PERCENTAGE DISTRIBUTION OF MARITAL STATUS
BY RACE AND HEALTH INSURANCE STATUS
NEW YORK CITY   RECORDED 1985

	UNWED	WED	TOTAL
NON HISPANIC WHITES			
MEDICAID	1,496 (42.5%)	2,022 (57.5%)	3,518 (100%)
THIRD PARTY INSURANCE	1,749 (5.5%)	30,293 (94.5%)	32,042 (100%)
NON HISPANIC BLACKS			
MEDICAID	15,530 (83.2%)	3,147 (16.8%)	18,677 (100%)
THIRD PARTY INSURANCE	5,607 (39.4%)	8,624 (60.6%)	14,231 (100%)
HISPANIC			
MEDICAID	11,874 (64.8%)	6,452 (35.2%)	18,326 (100%)
THIRD PARTY INSURANCE	2,930 (26.4%)	8,186 (73.6%)	11,116 (100%)

are unintended, it appears unlikely that teenagers seek pregnancy as a way to qualify for welfare benefits. Once pregnant, however, it is possible that the teenager's choice of pregnancy resolution is affected by the relative availability of welfare support; whether they remain at home or choose to live independently may have an important bearing on the likelihood of their finishing school (Bane & Ellwood, 1984). These and other potential associations between welfare and teenage childbearing pose very difficult cause-and-effect relationships that are presently unclear.

TABLE 6
PERCENTAGE DISTRIBUTION OF MARITAL STATUS
BY RACE AND SOCIO-ECONOMIC STATUS
UPSTATE NEW YORK RESIDENTS 1985

	UNWED	WED	TOTAL
NON HISPANIC WHITES			
LOW SES AREAS	2,407 (28.8%)	5,961 (71.2%)	8,368 (100%)
OTHER SES AREAS	13,769 (12.0%)	101,023 (88.0%)	114,792 (100%)
NON HISPANIC BLACKS			
LOW SES AREAS	3,402 (76.0%)	1,073 (24.0%)	4,475 (100%)
OTHER SES AREAS	4,953 (60.2%)	3,271 (39.8%)	8,224 (100%)
HISPANIC			
LOW SES AREAS	462 (51.2%)	441 (48.8%)	903 (100%)
OTHER SES AREAS	1,232 (29.7%)	2,916 (70.3%)	4,148 (100%)

On the subject of women and poverty, and the effects on reproductive status, a few other specific relationships are more clear, and discussion of each follows.

FAMILY PLANNING

Family planning implies conscious planning and appropriate actions to have or not have a child. Yet, many teenagers delay their first visit to a family planning clinic until a year or more after starting intercourse for fear that parents will find out (Zabin & Clark, 1981). While the estimated intended fertility in teenagers 15-19 in New York State in 1980 had dropped to 9.7 per 1000, from 21.1 per 1000 in 1974, the actual fertility dropped only 4.6 percentage points between 1974 and 1980, from 39.4 to 34.8 per 1000 (US DHEW Teenage Fertility, 1978 and, US DHHS, Selected Tables, Teenage Pregnancy and Fertility, 1986 — see Table 7).

The occurrence of pregnancy, planned or unplanned, has also been greatly influenced by recent trends such as changes in mari-

TABLE 7
DISTRIBUTION OF FEMALE VENEREAL DISEASE
CASES WITHIN CENSUS TRACT COUNTIES, 1985

Census Tract Status*	Early Syphilis	Percent	Uncomplicated Gonorrhea	Percent	GPID	Percent
Upper	27	20	605	11	69	10
Middle	51	38	1,204	22	176	25
Lower	51	38	3,418	63	437	62
Unknown	5	4	159	3	23	3
TOTAL	134	100	5,386	100	705	100
Total Upstate Cases Among Females	200		8,020		976	
Percent of cases located in scored census tracts	67		67		72	

*Based upon socioeconomic data (median household income, level of education, level of skilled labor) obtained by the 1980 Federal Census. Census tracts in the following counties have been scored on a scale of 1-12: Albany, Erie, Broome, Monroe, Nassau, Niagara, Oneida, Onondaga, Saratoga, Westchester. Scores of 0-4 are rated as lower class tracts; 5-9, middle; and 10-12, upper.

- - - - - - - -
Data supplied by the New York State Department of Health, Bureau of Communicable Disease Control, Sexually Transmitted Disease Control Program.

tal patterns, especially delayed marriage, increased divorce, and premarital intercourse (Pratt et al., 1984). Younger ages at first birth are strongly associated with subsequent higher overall fertility, more out-of-wedlock births and higher proportions of unwanted children (Moore & Burt, 1982). Women with less than 12 years of schooling have more children than those with more years of schooling. National fertility studies show that married women who have not finished high school have a higher proportion of recent unwanted births than those with more education. Many intermediate variables affect fertility, and contraception may be the most important one in the United States (Pratt et al., 1984), since with the increased early premarital exposure to sexual intercourse, early contraceptive use obviously has an important bearing on whether premarital pregnancy occurs. Utilization of family planning services is closely linked with contraceptive practice. Women with less than 12 years of schooling use publicly subsidized clinics more frequently than private physicians or counselors for family planning services (Pratt et al., 1984). A study of sources of family-planning visits for women ages 15-24 indicated that 50 percent made their first visit to a clinic. Black women were far more likely to use a clinic for their first visit than white women (72 percent vs. 45 percent) and for black women, the percentage using a clinic was highest for those with incomes below the poverty level, and those in the lowest education group (Mosher & Horn, 1986). Generally, very young and older mothers are overrepresented in populations from low socioeconomic levels (Hodgman, 1982). This holds true for New York State, although there are some ethnic variations. The distribution of total previous pregnancies among women delivering a live birth in 1985 shows a higher percentage of white women and Hispanic women who are poor having four or more pregnancies. Among Upstate black women, the percentage of births to women gravida four or higher is essentially the same for poor as for nonpoor. In New York City, poor black women have a lower percentage of gravida four or more than do the nonpoor (New York State Department of Health, Bureau of Biostatistics, 1986).

Statistics from family planning clinics (New York State Department of Health, Bureau of Reproductive Health, 1986) covering over 233,000 women, reflect this relationship between poverty, as represented by eligibility for Medicaid, pregnancy at an early or later age, higher fertility and lower educational attainment. Among the poor, the proportion of females under 15 was twice as high, and the proportion of females over 25 was one-third higher than for the comparable group who were not receiving medical assistance (2.9 percent vs. 1.4 percent, and 34.7 percent vs. 25.2 percent). Three-quarters of the poor already had a live birth, and only 15 percent had no previous pregnancy, compared to less than one-third (32.7 percent and 44.2 percent, respectively) among the non-Medicaid patients. Almost 27 percent of the poor had not completed high school, compared with only 15 percent of the group not receiving medical assistance. Only 12.5 percent had been to college, compared to one-third among the non-medical assistance group. The greatest difference was evident in the age group 18 to 19 with respect to prior pregnancies: among the Medicaid group, fully 70.1 percent had at least one pregnancy, whereas among the non-medical assistance group only 35 percent had a previous pregnancy.

Medicaid provides services only to a specific group of poor women — generally those on welfare — who have certain social characteristics and who also meet stringent income criteria. As a result, Medicaid's target population includes only about 33 percent of those low-income women the national family planning program seeks to reach. Almost all women eligible for Medicaid already have children and do not live with a spouse. In contrast, a large portion of the low-income women in need of family planning services and served by family-planning clinics either have no children or are married and living with their spouses; therefore, they are ineligible for Medicaid (Orr, 1981). In 1979, of women at risk of unintended pregnancy, only 63 percent of low or marginal-income women, and only 56 percent of 15-19 year olds, received medically supervised family-planning services (Torres et al., 1981).

The extent to which Medicaid subsidizes family planning services was examined in a 1982 study of the National Survey of Family Growth (NSFG). Only 30 percent of black teenagers, 18 percent of Hispanics, and 8 percent of whites were covered by Medicaid (Torres & Singh, 1986). In 1983, a higher proportion of each ethnic group was defined as poor — 33.7 percent of blacks, 28.4 percent of Hispanics, and 12.1 percent of whites (O'Hare, 1985)—and at some time these newly poor young women will need subsidized services as they will be at higher risk of unintended pregnancies because of limited access to care. Ironically, it appears that poverty means limited access to the very services that help to prevent poverty.

On the other hand, family planning programs that serve poor women have not always been viewed as operating in the best interest of these women. As late as 1985, Thomas Shapiro wrote,

> In the 1970s there was a dramatic increase in the use of sterilization as a method of contraception. Female sterilization is the most rapidly growing form of birth control in the United States, rising from 200,000 cases in 1970 to over 700,000 in 1980.

He observed that funds for sterilization became accessible officially in 1971, making this method of contraception widely available for poor women in a decade when there were drastic cutbacks in virtually all other public services. It was also a decade during which abortions became legal, yet were severely restricted for the poor. In his view, our population policies during the 1970s functioned systemically to target poor women, especially those on welfare, for fertility control. His thesis, "the use of contraceptive devices varies according to class, gender, and race; and, broad social conditions, cultural traditions, and structural inequalities play a large part in shaping a woman's birth control experience," reaffirms the connection between women, poverty, and reproductive status. Female sterilization, controversial, risky, irreversible, and federally financed for the poor, was at one time in our history the birth control method that was often recommended for poor women.

SEXUALLY TRANSMISSIBLE DISEASES AND ECTOPIC PREGNANCIES

The term sexually transmissible diseases (STD) represents a shift in terminology due to an increased awareness that many infectious diseases are transmissible through sexual contact as well as an increased diversity of such diseases.

Women, and especially the poor, are disproportionately affected by the medical complications associated with sexually transmissible diseases. Recent estimates suggest that 2.6 million women are infected each year in the United States with *Chlamydia trachomatis*. Although these numbers are in themselves staggering, it is the serious complications of chlamydial infection in women and children that are of greatest concern to public health officials (Mason, 1986). Poor women, due to limited access to adequate medical care, are impacted most heavily by the complications associated with chlamydia, such as urethritis, cervicitis, and pelvic inflammatory disease. It is estimated that gonorrhea and chlamydia are responsible for almost 80 percent of the pelvic inflammatory disease (PID) seen in hospital emergency rooms each year. Infection resulting in acute pelvic inflammatory disease increases a woman's risk for ectopic pregnancy, and the risk of infertility increase sevenfold after one episode of PID. National experts fear that chlamydia infections are epidemic, yet those infections are not well-recognized and often not often well-treated (Holmes, 1981).

The impact of STDs on poor women extends beyond their own personal health to that of their children. Infants acquire chlamydial and gonococcal infections at birth from contact with infected cervical and vaginal secretions of their mothers. Nearly 10 percent of pregnant women in the United States will be infected with *C. trachomatis* resulting in some 120,000 infants contracting chlamydia infections. Chlamydia is the most common cause of neonatal eye infection, leading to an estimated 74,000 cases of inclusion conjunctivitis annually. Afebrile interstitial pneumonia in infants under three months of age is caused most frequently by *C. trachomatis* than by any other organism; approximately 37,000 cases of chlamydia pneumonia occur each year (Mason, 1986). Other conditions, though they occur less frequently, are devastating to the child and the family involved. Neonatal gonorrhea infection has decreased, but only as a result of a law that requires the application of prophylactic antibiotics to the conjunctiva of newborns.

The newest and potentially most serious STD is Acquired Immuno-Deficiency Syndrome (AIDS). While AIDS or its caus-ative agent is not yet highly prevalent among women in this country, there is some evidence that this trend is changing. In Africa, women comprise 47-50 percent of the total number of AIDS cases (Ebbeson, 1984). In the United States, women ac-count for 6.6 percent of known AIDS cases (Centers for Disease Control, AIDS Weekly, 1986). At the present time, reported cases of AIDS in women in New York State account for 9.8 percent of adult cases, and seem to occur in economically de-pressed areas.

In New York City, AIDS is the leading cause of death for women between the ages of 25-29 (Lower East Side Study, Stuy-vesant Clinic, 1986). While data on humans immuno-virus (HIV) seroprevalence are incomplete, the existing data indicate high rates of HIV infection in women or in their male partners. The number of black and Hispanic women affected by AIDS/ HIV infection is disproportionately high (New York State De-partment of Health, AIDS Institute, 1986).

There are similarities between the incidence of unplanned pregnancy and STDs. Both conditions are "biologically sexist": women usually bear the greater health risks and potential repro-ductive consequences of both. Low-income patients in urban ar-eas are more likely to have unplanned pregnancies or STDs, and young inner-city blacks are at greater risk for both (Hatcher, 1986). Women usually develop more severe cases of genital her-pes initially, and these women run a fourfold greater risk of cer-vical cancer than women who have not contracted herpes (US DHHS, Women's Health, 1985).

MATERNAL DEATHS

A maternal death is also "sexist" and is the quintessence of Freud's statement that biology is destiny; it can only happen to a woman. Ectopic pregnancies are related to PIDs and STDs, both of which occur more often in low-socioeconomic groups. The number of reported ectopic pregnancies tripled from 17,800 in 1970 to 52,000 in 1980 and the rate among total pregnancies doubled in the United States. As a result, ectopic pregnancies are now the leading cause of maternal death during the first three months of pregnancy, and the leading cause of maternal deaths among black women (US DHHS, Women's Health, 1985).

Another contributor to maternal mortality is cesarean childbirth, the incidence of which has increased from 16.5 percent in 1980 to approximately 18.5 percent in 1982 (US DHHS, Women's Health, 1985), and the maternal morbidity rate for women having cesarean sections is 12 times that for vaginal deliveries (Nielsen, 1986). In a study of maternal deaths that occurred during the five year period 1974-1978, epidemiologists from the U.S. Centers for Disease Control (CDC) found that embolism, hypertensive disease, and obstetric hemorrhage led the list of causes of death associated with live births; ectopic pregnancies, and all types of abortions led the list in pregnancies not ending in live births (Kaunitz, 1985). Seifert and Doss-Martin reported on a study conducted at the University of Michigan (1986) which showed that black women in the United States were three times as likely as white women to die in childbirth, generally because of their poor living conditions and inadequate access to prenatal care (N.Y. Amsterdam News, 8/26/86).

CERVICAL CANCER

The relationship of the incidence of cervical cancer, mortality and survival with poverty status has been recognized for some time. Among the classical formal studies of this relationship are those of Clemmesen and Nielsen (1951). In Copenhagen, the age-adjusted incidence of cervical cancer was seen to increase with declining social class as measured by the average house rent of the subdistrict of residence. In the work by Logan (1954) on England and Wales, standardized cervical cancer mortality ratios for married women were found to be greater in the lower social classes as indicated by occupation of the husband. In the United States, Graham et al. (1960) found cervical cancer incidence in white women in Buffalo, N.Y. to increase with decreasing median rental value of the census tract of residence, and Lundin et al. (1964) showed the incidence in white women in a cytological screening program in Memphis to increase with declining socioeconomic status as measured by male occupational distribution in the census tract of residence as well as by educational level, rent and level of residential crowding. Rotkin and Cameron (1968) found clusters of economic and sociological variables to be significant correlates of cervical cancer incidence.

In more recent studies, the inverse relationship between cervical cancer incidence and social class was observed in Cali, Columbia (Cuello et al., 1982), where social class was determined according to census tract of residence, and in New Jersey (Najeem & Greer, 1985), where socioeconomic status was measured by per capita income. In Finland, cervical cancer incidence has been found to be inversely associated with individual occupation and education, although incidence rates were directly correlated with a standard living index derived from municipalities. Data from the Third National Cancer Survey (Devesa, 1984) show negative associations of cervical cancer incidence with income and education derived from census tract of residence among both blacks and whites.

While cervical cancer incidence among Hispanics is lower than that for blacks, American Indians and Chinese-Americans, and higher than in whites, the incidence of cervical cancer is twice as high among Hispanics in New Mexico and Puerto Rico as in nonminorities there (US DHHS, Report of the Secretary's Task Force on Black and Minority Health, Vol. 3). New York State Cancer Registry data also show cervical cancer incidence and mortality in New York City to be substantially higher among blacks than among whites, with Hispanics occupying an intermediate position (see Figure 1). Cancer incidence rates for New York State reflect this trend as well (see Table 8).

Much of the observed excess risk for minority women is probably accounted for by differences in socioeconomic distribution; when socioeconomic distribution was adjusted for in Third National Cancer Survey data, the excess in cervical cancer risk for blacks compared to whites was reduced from more than 70 percent to less than 30 percent (Devesa, 1984).

Sociodemographic status is an indication of a whole spectrum of lifestyle factors in addition to the material and intellectual quality of life (as measured by income and education). Social

Figure 1

CANCER INCIDENCE IN NEW YORK CITY 1978 - 1982
AGE ADJUSTED RATES*FOR ETHNIC GROUPS
Site Cervix Uteri (180)

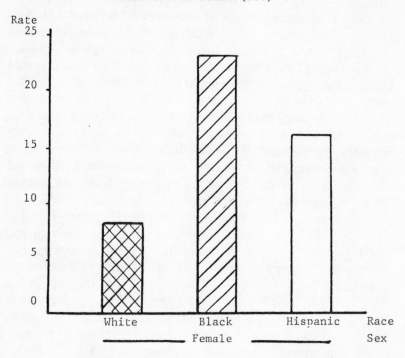

* Per 100,000 - Adjusted to 1970 U.S. Population

patterns and practices differ as well, and early on in the study of
cervical cancer it was realized that cervical cancer incidence varied with a woman's marital status and age at first marriage. Subsequent studies revealed that these associations could be accounted for by the number of sexual partners and age at first
intercourse. These associations can be explained by an infectious
disease model of cervical cancer in which the adolescent cervix
may be more susceptible to infection and the risk of infection
increases with the number of sexual partners. Studies of hus-

TABLE 8
NEW YORK STATE DEPARTMENT OF HEALTH
CANCER REGISTRY
AGE ADJUSTED* AND AVERAGE ANNUAL CANCER INCIDENCE
RATES PER 100,000 BY RACE AND SEX SELECTED SITES
NEW YORK STATE 1978-1982

| | MALES | | | FEMALES | | |
	WHITE[1]	BLACK	OTHER	WHITE[1]	BLACK	OTHER
All Malignant Neoplasms (140-208)**	391.2	448.6	232.8	309.1	279.0	156.7
Lip, oral cavity and pharynx (140-149)	14.4	22.8	13.4	5.5	6.5	4.3
Esophagus (150)	5.6	22.7	4.6	1.9	5.9	1.4
Stomach (151)	13.3	22.2	17.2	6.6	10.8	8.7
Colon (153)	45.4	39.1	26.1	34.5	32.0	15.8
Rectum (154)	21.7	14.3	15.6	13.2	11.0	6.1
Pancreas (157)	12.5	15.2	6.4	8.6	10.6	3.9
Layrnx (161)	9.7	12.2	2.7	1.8	2.0	0.1
Trachea, bronchus, and lung (162)	80.5	102.5	48.1	28.6	26.3	17.6
Malignant melanoma of skin (172)	7.6	0.8	0.8	6.0	0.9	0.8
Female breast (174)	-	-	-	86.2	66.3	34.6
Uterus, except cervix (179, 182)	-	-	-	21.4	13.1	7.6
Cervix uteri - invasive (180)	-	-	-	9.2	21.3	12.6
Ovary and other uterine adnexa (183)	-	-	-	15.0	9.9	6.8
Prostate (185)	58.5	102.6	20.4	-	-	-
Testis (186)	4.0	0.7	1.0	-	-	-
Bladder (188)	32.4	13.8	11.9	8.3	5.9	2.5
Kidney, etc. (189)	10.4	8.2	5.5	NA	NA	NA
Thyroid gland (193)	2.1	0.8	1.9	4.2	2.5	3.9
Lymphoma (200-202)	17.0	10.5	8.1	12.5	7.1	3.2
Leukemia (204-208)	12.7	8.6	10.4	7.9	6.1	4.2
Cervix uteri-in situ (233.1)	-	-	-	20.8	34.4	16.5

* Adjusted to Census of U.S. 1970.
** ICD 9th, 1975

[1]White - Cases with race unknown (2.16% of total) included as white because
more than 85% of these unknowns occurred in the geographic area
outside New York City where the population is predominantly white.

- Denominators for the calculation of rates include Spanish origin not
specified as Black. In the Census of 1980, the Spanish origin
population in New York State was counted:

White	796	134	(48.0%)
Black	102	879	(6.2%)
Other races	760	287	(45.8%)
Total	1659	300	

that is, 45.8% of the Spanish origin population was listed as neither
white nor black. We believe most of these are Puerto Rican and should
be considered white.

bands of women with cervical cancer which have shown the husbands to have greater numbers of sex partners (Buckley et al., 1981; Zunzunequi et al., 1986) also support this model, and certain viruses are under investigation as potential disease agents.

In the face of this evidence it is significant that the cervical cancer-poverty association persists even when reproductive factors are controlled for. The effect of socioeconomic status thus cannot be due entirely to reproductive behavior, and some additional mechanism must be sought.

Another factor related to socioeconomic status that has also been related to cervical cancer is cigarette smoking (Williams & Horm, 1977). Cervical cancer incidence tends to be higher in smokers, however it is unclear whether this association represents a truly causal relationship or merely reflects the greater prevalence of cigarette smoking among members of a group already at higher risk due to other social and behavioral factors.

CONCLUSION

There is a connection between poverty and reproductive status in women, with health status declining as socioeconomic status, including income, declines. Because women are disproportionately represented among the poor, they are at risk for poor health, particularly poor reproductive status. The health gap between poor and nonpoor people is related to the absence of financial and other resources that afford access to health and medical care. The long-term effects of the poverty syndrome, which leads to chronic low-socioeconomic status, reinforces this deficiency in access to services, so the poor get poorer and sicker. The health gap for poor women is significant to the larger society since the health status of women directly affects the health status of future generations. Therefore, there needs to be a renewed ideological commitment to reproductive health care for women that transcends notions of race and class. The often-repeated statement "health care is a right" should be enforced through a new social contract between women and the state that enables women to exercise this right to health care within reason, and without the unnecessary barriers that arise due to lack of financial resources and the presence of class biases.

RECOMMENDATIONS

1. Government-supported programs of health education and promotion should be targeted to poor women since much of the observed health gap is related to lifestyle and knowledge.

2. All women, regardless of socioeconomic status and age, should have guaranteed access to comprehensive health services; and, the right of access should be supported by a state-sponsored reimbursement system that does not in itself constitute a barrier to access.

3. The health services provided to women should include periodic health assessment, including screening for disease of the reproductive system, and the capacity for case management to keep poor women in the system.

4. Health programs should acknowledge cultural and ethnic differences among women, and programs should be designed and professional and other staff selected, with these issues that present barriers to utilization of health services, in mind.

5. The system of public assistance should address the range of human needs, including housing quality and quantity, nutrition, and education, which are contributors to low socioeconomic status.

NOTES

1. New York State Department of Health (1986) Bureau of Biostatistics. For this paper, the Bureau reviewed selected reproductive health outcome data, as follows:

Certificates of live births for 1985 were used as an additional data source in investigating the impact of poverty on reproductive status. The analysis is segregated into two distinct sections (1) events occurring in New York City and, (2) events occurring in Upstate New York. The New York City certificates contain information on financial coverage and those live births covered by Medicaid are contrasted with other third party coverage as a means of comparing outcomes between poor and nonpoor women. For the purpose of this analysis, self-pay, live births are excluded due to ambiguity in classifying such events according to poverty status.

For live births occurring in Upstate New York, the outcomes for women residing in

low socioeconomic areas are compared outcomes for women residing in the remainder
of New York State. The areas are classified according to a composite socioeconomic
score, based on information from the 1980 U.S. Census. The composite score considers
median family income, percent unskilled workers among employed persons at least 10
years of age.

The Mantel-Haenszel statistic is used to calculate an adjusted odds ratio across the
three population categories: non-Hispanic white, non-Hispanic black, and Hispanic.
The odds ratio provides a summary measure of the differential levels of outcome considered.

REFERENCES

Alan Guttmacher Institute, (1985). Paying for maternity care. *Family Planning Perspectives, 17*(3), May-June, 103-11.
Bane, M. J. & Ellwood, D. T. (1983). *The dynamics of dependence: the routes to self
sufficiency,* Cambridge, MA, Harvard University, as cited in Ellwood, "Report of
the Proceedings of the Public Assistance Employment Conference," Saratoga
Springs, NY, Nov. 3-4, 1983, pp. 40-55.
Buckley, J. D., Harris, R. W. C., Doll, R. et al. (1981). Case-control study of the
husbands of women with dysplasia or carcinoma of the cervix uteri. *Lancet, ii,*
1010.
Centers for Disease Control (1986). *AIDS Weekly,* June 16.
Centers for Health Economics Research (1982). Access to ob-gyn services under Medi-
caid, Boston, Mass., Research Report.
Chilman, C. (1979). As cited in Moore, K. A. & Burt, M. R., q.v.p. 44.
Clemmesen, J. & Nielsen, A. (1951). The social distribution of cancer in Copenhagen.
British Journal of Cancer, 5, 159-171.
C. S. Mott Foundation (1986). *Teenage pregnancy: An update and guide to Mott Foun-
dation Resources,* Flint, Michigan.
Cuello, C., Correa, P. & Haenszel, W. (1982). Socio-economic class differences in
cancer incidence in Cali, Columbia. *International Journal of Cancer, 29,* 637-643.
Davis, C. Haub, C. & Willette, J. (1983). U.S. Hispanic: Changing the face of Amer-
ica. *Population Bulletin, 38*(3).
Devesa, S. S. (1984). Descriptive epidemiology of cancer of the uterine cervix. *Obstet-
rics and Gynecology, 61,* 605-612.
Dorn, H. F. & Cutler, S. J. (1959). *Morbidity from cancer in the U.S.,* Public Health
Service, Publication No. 590. Washington, DC: U.S. Government Printing Office.
As cited in Kane, Kasteler & Gray, 1976, *The Health Gap.* New York: Springer
Publishing Co.
Ebbsen, P. (ed.) (1984). *AIDS.* Philadelphia: Saunders Co. Philadelphia.
Ehrenreich, B. & Piven, F. F. (1984). The feminization of poverty. *Dissent, 31,* 2,
Spring, 102.
Ellis, J. M. (1958). *Socio-economic differentials in mortality from chronic disease, in
patients, physicians, and illness,* E. Gartley Jaco, ed. (New York: Free Press), pp.
30-37.
Ford K. (1983). Second pregnancies among teenage mothers. *Family Planning Per-
spectives, 15*(6), pp. 262-278.
Graham, S., Levin, M. & Lilienfeld, A. M., (1960). The socio-economic distribution
of cancer in various sites in Buffalo, N.Y., 1948-1952. *Cancer, 13*(1), 180-191.

Greene, C. R. (1970). Medical care for underprivileged populations. *New England Journal of Medicine, 282*:1187-93.

Hakama, M. et al. (1982). Risk indicators of breast and cervical cancer in ecologic and individual levels. *American Journal of Epidemiology, 116,* 990-1000.

Harrington, M. (1984). *The new American poverty.* New York: Basic Books.

Hatcher, R. A. et al. (1986). *Contraceptive technology, 1986-1987.* New York: Irvington Publishers.

Hodgman, J. E. (1982). Pregnancy outcome, neonatal mortality and long-term morbidity. *Women: A developmental perspective.* U.S. Department of Health and Human Services, Public Health Service, National Institutes of Health, pp. 259-263.

Holmes, K. K., (1981). The chlamydia epidemic. *Journal of the American Medical Association, 245,* 17, 1718-1723.

Kane, R. L., Kasteler, J. M. & Gray, R. M., eds. (1976). *The health gap: medical services and the poor.* New York: Springer Publishing Co. p. 3.

Kaunitz, A. M. (1985). Causes of maternal mortality in the United States. *Journal of the American College of Obstetricians and Gynecologists, 65*:605. As cited in *Family Planning Perspectives, 17*(6), 270-271.

Kessner, D. M. et al., (1973). *Infant death: An analysis of maternal risk and health care.* Washington, DC: National Academy of Sciences.

Logan, W. P. D. (1954). Social class variations in mortality. *Public Health Reports, 69,* 1217-1223.

Lower East Side Study (1986). New York City: Stuyvesant Clinic.

Lundin, F. E. et al. (1964). Socio-economic distribution of cervical cancer—in relation to early marriage and pregnancy. Public Health Monograph, no. 73.

Mason, L. O. *Statement before the Subcommittee on Health and the Environment,* Committee on Energy and Commerce, U.S. House of Representatives, May 19, 1986, Centers for Disease Control, Atlanta, GA.

McLaughlin, S. D. et al. (1986). The effects of sequencing of marriage and first births during adolescence. *Family Planning Perspectives, 18*(1), 12-18.

Moore, K. & Waite, L. J. (1977). Early childbearing and educational attainment. *Family Planning Perspectives, 9,* 220-225.

Moore, K. A. & Burt, M. R. (1982). *Private crisis, public cost: Policy perspectives on teenage childbearing.* Washington, DC: The Urban Institute Press.

Mosher, W. D. & Horn, M. C., (1986). Source of service and visit rate of family planning services: United States, 1982. *Public Health Reports, 101*(4), pp. 405-416.

Mott, F. L. & Marsiglio, W. (1985). Early childbearing and completion of high school. *Family Planning Perspectives, 18*(1), 5-12.

Murray, C. (1984). *Losing ground: American social policy 1950-1980.* New York, Basic Books.

Najem, G. R. & Greer, T. W. (1985). Female reproductive organs and breast cancer mortality in New Jersey counties and the relationship with certain environmental variables. *Preventive Medicine, 14,* 620-635.

Newell, K. W. (1975). Global strategies—developing a unified strategy. *Oxford Textbook of Public Health, 2,* History, determinants, scope, and strategies. New York: Oxford University Press, p. 261.

New York Amsterdam News, August 16, 1986. Report on the work by Seifert and Doss-Martin (1986) U. of Michigan.

New York State Department of Health (1986). Communication from the AIDS Institute.

New York State Department of Health (1985). *Fiscal year 1986/87* Expenditure Plan, Bureau of Reproductive Health.

New York State Department of Health (1986). *New York State Family Planning Data System*, special run, Bureau of Reproductive Health.

New York State Department of Labor (1986). *Statistics relating to women and the labor force, earnings and poverty with emphasis on recent data*. DeSantis, V. et al.

New York Times, August 11, 1985.

New York Times, September 10, 1986, Book Review.

New York Times, September 25, 1986, Editorial.

O'Hare, W. P. (1985). Poverty in America: Trends and new patterns. *Population Bulletin, 40*(3).

Orr, M. T. & Brenner, L. (1981). Medicaid funding of family planning clinic services. *Family Planning Perspectives, 13*(6), 280-87.

Otten, A. (1985). Decision makers often fail to spot key changes behind the statistics. *Wall Street Journal*, December 6.

Pearce, D. & McAdoo, H. (1981). *Women and children: alone and in poverty*. Washington, DC: National Advisory Council on Economic Opportunity.

Pratt, W. F. et al. (1984). Understanding U.S. fertility: Findings from the national survey of family growth, cycle 111. *Population Bulletin, 39*(5).

Reid, J. (1982). Black America in the 1980s. *Population Bulletin, 37*(4).

Rotkin, I. D. & Cameron, J. R., Jr. (1968). Clusters of variables influencing risk of cervical cancer. *Cancer, 21*, 663-671.

Shapiro, T. M. (1985). *Population control politics: Women, sterilization, and reproductive choice*. Philadelphia: Temple University Press, pp. 6, 9, 25.

Thorton, A. & Freeman, D. (1983). The changing American family. *Population Bulletin, 38*(4).

Torres, A. & Forrest, J. D. (1983). Family planning clinic services in the United States, 1981. *Family Planning Perspectives, 15*(6), 272-78.

Torres et al. (1981). Family planning services in the United States, 1978-79. *Family Planning Perspectives, 13*(3), 132-141.

Torres, A, & Singh, S. (1986). Contraceptive practice among Hispanic adolescents. *Family Planning Perspectives, 18*(4), 193-94.

U.S. Department of Health, Education and Welfare, Public Health Service (1973). Limitations of activities due to chronic conditions, U.S., 1969 and 1970. *Vital and Health Statistics*, Series 10, No. 80, Washington DC: U.S. Government Printing Office.

U.S. Department of Health Education, and Welfare (1968). *Human investment program: Delivery of health services for the poor*, Washington, DC: U.S. Government Printing Office.

U.S. Department of Health, Education and Welfare, Public Health Service (1973). Mortality trends: Age, color and sex, U.S., 1950-69. National Health Survey, *Vital and Health Statistics*, Series 20, No. 15. Washington DC: U.S. Government Printing Office.

U.S. Department of Health Education and Welfare, Public Health Service (1978). *Teenage fertility in the United States*, Centers for Disease Control.

U.S. Department of Health and Human Services, Public Health Service (1985). *Health Status of Minorities and Low Income Groups*.

U.S. Department of Health and Human Services (1986). *Report of the Secretary's Task Force on Black and Minority Health*, Vol. VI. Infant mortality and low birth weight.

U.S. Department of Health and Human Services, Public Health Service (1986). *Selected tables, teenage pregnancy and fertility, U.S., 1974-1980*, Centers for Disease Control, Table 7. (Prerelease to State Health Agencies, 1986).

U.S. Department of Health and Human Services, Public Health Service (1982). National Center for Health Statistics, *Dietary intake data*, 1976-1980. Series 11, No. 231.

Verbrugge, L. M. (1979). Marital status and health. *Marriage and Family*, *42*, 267-285.

Wall Street Journal, August 27, 1986.

White, E. L. (1986). A graphic presentation of age and income differentials in selected aspects of morbidity, disability, and utilization of health services. *Inquiry*, *5*, 18-30.

William R. R. & Horm, J. W. (1977). Association of cancer sites with tobacco and alcohol consumption and socioeconomic status of patients: Interview study from the Third National Cancer Survey. *Junci*, *58*(3), 525-547.

Zabin, S. & Clark, S. D., Jr. Why they delay: A study of teenage family planning clinic patients. *Family Planning Perspectives*, *13*(5), 205-217.

Zunzunequi, M. V., King, M. C., Coria, C. F. & Charlet, J. (1986). Male influences on cervical cancer risk. *AM J. Epidemiology*, *123*, 302-307.

The Working Environment
of the Working Poor:
An Analysis Based on Workers'
Compensation Claims, Census Data
and Known Risk Factors

Jeanne Mager Stellman, PhD

SUMMARY. Analysis of 1980 U.S. Census data reveals that a sizeable percentage of adult females employed full-time (working more than 2080 hours in 1979) worked in female-dominated service, sales and factory occupations and had family incomes which placed them in poverty or impoverishment status. Workers' compensation data on women in these occupations, drawn from the 27-state Supplemental Data System, show that they filed approximately 250,000 claims for compensation in 1980. Analysis of the claims by nature of injury and body part affected is consistent with the published medical literature. Injury to the back is the leading complaint filed and large numbers of hand and wrist injuries are also reported.

Compensation data, however, are usually reflective of acute conditions, especially traumatic injury, not of chronic illnesses and injuries. Additional data are therefore drawn from the medical and scientific literature. This review shows the presence of cancer-causing agents, infectious agents, reproductive toxins, safety hazards and social stressors in these occupations. Recommendations for future programs and needs are presented.

Jeanne Mager Stellman is Associate Professor, School of Public Health, Columbia University, and is affiliated with the Women's Occupational Health Resource Center. Reprint requests may be addressed to The Women's Occupational Health Resource Center, 117 St. John's Place, Brooklyn, NY 11217.

INTRODUCTION

Social action and social legislation based on concern about the health and well-being of poor and powerless women in the workplace has been called the "driving wedge" for modern labor legislation. Such social action led to establishing the first regulations of working conditions (Brandeis, 1918). It was for women that the laws setting a maximum number of hours of work per day were first passed and successfully withstood the tests of the courts. The United States Supreme Court upheld the constitutionality of an Oregon maximum hours of work law in 1908 (*Muller* v. *Oregon*, 1908) although it had set aside a similar New York law several years earlier. Women, in the Court's written opinion in the Oregon case, were explicitly more fragile and hence more in need of protection than men. Therefore special protective rules, which would otherwise have been considered by the Court to be an infringement of the rights of free enterprise when applied to men, could be justified and established for females.

In the same social vein of protection of females and, ipso facto "of the species" (as the Supreme Court decision stated in 1908), minimum wage laws for women and children were promulgated, and only later, extended to men. The early part of the twentieth century saw the passage of the first "protective" laws for women workers by which females were specifically prohibited from workplaces where particular toxic substances, such as lead or benzene, were used. They were prohibited from working in mines, lifting loads beyond a certain weight and working at night, except for women in certain exempted "female" jobs such as nursing. Although these "protective" laws have since been found to be discriminatory against women and have been struck down in the United States, as well as in some other countries where women's rights movements have become established, they are still in effect in many countries and incorporated in international standards-setting organizations, like the International Labour Office (Ratner, 1980; Hunt, 1979).

Given this early legislative and social consciousness about the risks of adverse occupational exposures on the health of women workers, one might conjecture that the occupational environment in female-dominated trades should present few hazards, a low rate of accidents, injuries and illnesses and adequate compensation. However, an examination of the working environment of the majority of women workers in the United States in 1986, some four score years after the upholding of *Muller* v. *Oregon* by the U.S. Supreme Court, does not support this conjecture. In fact, the data show that the majority of women workers are in occupations in which at least 10% of all full-time employed women workers are impoverished. And, concurrently, hundreds of thousands of women are injured on the job each year. Many toxic chemicals and dangerous working conditions can be present in jobs traditionally held by women and often considered "safe" (Hunt, 1979; Stellman, 1977; Chavkin, 1984). Rather than being protected and cared for, large numbers of female American workers are both economically disadvantaged, while being employed full-time, and also at risk for health hazards on the job.

In order to shed further light on the environmental working conditions of the working poor, this paper will explore data on the impoverishment of working women based on demographic information in the 1980 Census of the U.S. population and on the occupational health of working women using workers' compensation data collected by the U.S. Bureau of Labor Statistics' Supplemental Data System, a cooperative program between the U.S. Department of Labor and 27 states (U.S. Department of Labor, 1980). In the Supplemental Data System information on injury and illnesses from each participating state is coded and combined in compatible format.

In addition, general information on occupational hazards to women workers in these occupations is drawn from technical, medical and social literature. The analysis of these data sources shows that in 1980 there were a large number of women who suffered ill effects from occupational exposures, many in the same occupations in which large numbers of women are also laboring for wages that keep them in a state of poverty or impoverishment, particularly if they are young, with families and not married.

POVERTY AND WOMEN'S OCCUPATIONS

The 1980 census of population and housing provides a massive data base on earnings and occupations of residents of the United States. Using a subset of the data that is contained in the public-use microdata samples, PUMS (U.S. Department of Commerce, 1983), the occupation, family income and poverty status of a 0.1% sample of the total population base was extracted and data on women employed full-time during 1979 were analyzed. Full-time employment was defined as any job in which the product of weeks worked and hours worked equalled or exceeded 2080 during the calendar year. This cutoff was chosen because frequency analysis revealed it to be a clear demarcation between full-time and part-time workers. It appears that most workers characterized themselves as working 40 hours per week and 52 weeks per year, regardless of varying vacation and sick leave allotments.

Women who worked full-time were further characterized by the level at which their family income placed them with respect to the national norms for poverty. The Bureau of the Census has created a variable in the data set entitled POVERTY, which corresponds to the percentage of the defined levels of "poverty" represented by each individual's family income. Table 1 gives the poverty levels used in the 1980 Census. "Poverty" has been recoded in this paper into three strata: (1) at or below poverty level; (2) less than two times poverty; (3) more than two times the poverty level. I will concentrate the analyses and discussion on the two levels, (1) and (2), which I term "poverty" and "impoverishment," respectively, and corresponding to family income below the poverty level and family income less than two times the national poverty norms.

The population is also classified by marital status and race. All women who were not married at the time of the census are classified as "not married" and the group was divided into "white" and "non-white" racial categories. More detailed subdivisions for marital status or for non-white racial subgroup were not practical given the occupational dispersion of the group. A cross-tabulation of selected occupations of full-time employment by the two economic indices, "poverty" and "impoverishment," and by marital status and rate is given in Tables 2, 3a and 3b.

Examination of the data in Table 2 reveals that a large number of all employed women, married or unmarried, white or non-white, young or old, work full-time and still live at or below the poverty level. In some occupations, like building services or laundry work, 28% to 43% of unmarried non-white women un-

Table 1. Definitions of Poverty Level Thresholds in 1979 by Size of
Family and Number of Related Children Under 18 Years of Age, 1980 Census*

| Size of Family Unit | None | 1 | Number of Related Children Under 18 Years of Age | | | | | | | |
			2	3	4	5	6	7	8	9
1 person										
under 65 years	$3,774									
65 years & older	3,479									
2 persons										
householder under 65	4,858	5,000								
householder 65 & over	4,385	4,981								
3 persons	5,674	5,839	5,844							
4 persons	7,482	7,605	7,356	7,382						
5 persons	9,023	9,154	8,874	8,657	8,525					
6 persons	9,915	10,378	10,419	10,205	9,999	9,693	9,512			
7 persons	11,941	12,016	11,759	11,580	11,246	10,857	10,429			
8 persons	13,356	13,473	13,231	13,018	12,717	12,334	11,936	11,835		
9 or more persons	16,066	16,144	15,929	15,749	15,453	15,046	14,677	14,586	14,024	

* Taken from U.S.Department of Commerce (1983).

der the age of 45 are full-time poverty-stricken workers. In the textile industry approximately 10% of women under the age of 45, both white and non-white, will be poverty stricken. Being a full-time sewing machine operator means a life of poverty for one out of five non-white older married females.

More black women are impoverished than are white women. The unmarried woman worker is economically worse off than the married one. If one considers the occupational distribution of all black women, a full 71% of the occupations of black unmarried females are ones in which at least 13% of the workers are from impoverished families.

Analysis of impoverishment by age shows that older workers, defined as women over the age of 45, are generally more impoverished than younger workers, although there is some variation among the occupations. Tables 3a and 3b give the occupational distribution of the entire group according to age and the percentage who live in a state of impoverishment. Again, there is a disparity between white and non-white workers and married and unmarried workers, even in the same occupational groups. More non-whites are impoverished than whites and higher percentages of unmarried women of all races are impoverished.

Impoverishment is not bound by occupational class. Impoverished workers can be found among clerical and office workers, industrial and agricultural workers and workers in the service industries.

Table 2. Percent of Women in Selected Occupations Employed Full-Time And Living At or Below Poverty Level

Occupation	Married Whites	Married Non-white	Unmarried White	Unmarried Non-white
less than 45 years of age:				
Service				
Food services (prep)	5.4	3.8	7.5	17.2
Waitress/bartending	13.3	12.5	14.1	--
Personal services	1.9	15.1	15.1	23.1
Private household	16.7	25.0	20.0	16.6
Building services	5.9	4.2	14.0	28.1
Health Services	2.3	3.2	2.4	10.2
Retail Sales	1.7	3.8	4.5	4.6
Industry/Agriculture				
Agriculture/Forestry	10.5		14.8	20.0
Stitchers & Sewers	3.6	2.8	13.2	7.4
Laundry	--	14.3	14.3	42.9
Textiles	11.1	9.1	9.5	--
Machine op - asst'd	0.7	7.9	5.2	13.2
Fabricators,assemblers, handworking			5.3	8.1
Clerical/Office				
Office clerical	0.5	--	4.5	2.1
Data entry	--	4.5	--	--
Secretary/typist	0.6	0.9	1.2	4.0
Bookkeeping/related	1.5	--	2.4	3.2
45 years of age or older:				
Service				
Food services (prep)	--	17.2	18.1	14.3
Waitress/bartending	8.8	--	20.0	--
Personal services	5.9			14.3
Private household	12.5	10.0	12.9	
Building services	5.8	2.8	5.0	17.9
Health Services		3.2	3.0	5.2
Retail Sales	2.5		7.8	
Industry/Agriculture				
Agriculture/Forestry		16.7	7.7	
Stitchers & Sewers	1.6	22.2	7.2	11.1
Laundry	12.6	--	--	18.2
Machine op - asst'd	2.5	6.7	2.0	
Clerical/Office				
Office clerical	1.2			
Secretary/typist			1.0	9.1
Bookkeeping/related	0.5		2.3	

Source: U.S. Department of Commerce (1983)

Table 3a. Women in Selected Occupations Employed Full-Time
And Living in Impoverishment*: 45 Years of Age and Older

Occupation	Married				Unmarried			
	White		Non-white		White		Non-white	
	% impover-ished	% all jobs	% impover-ished	% all jobs	% impover-ished	% all jobs	% impover-ished	% all jobs
Service								
Food services (prep)	14.8	2.0	13.5	6.2	42.6	3.5	38.2	6.2
Waitress/bartending	23.5	1.3	40.0	1.4	53.0	1.0	42.9	2.1
Personal services	11.8	0.6	30.0	2.8	56.3	0.9	28.5	4.1
Cosmetology/barber	6.7	0.6	100.0	0.3	18.2	0.6	50.0	1.2
Private household	37.5	0.3	30.3	2.8	68.1	1.8	75.1	7.1
Building services	17.4	1.9	8.4	10.1	25.0	2.3	39.9	11.5
Health Services	10.8	3.4	22.6	8.7	30.9	3.9	34.3	11.7
Retail Sales	7.6	5.9	--.	1.7	25.4	5.8	20.0	1.5
Industry/Agriculture								
Agriculture/Forestry	23.1	2.1	16.7	1.7	24.6	0.7	--	
Stitchers & Sewers	12.8	2.5	33.3	2.6	28.6	1.7	44.4	2.7
Laundry	18.9	0.6	42.9	2.1	41.6	0.7	36.4	3.3
Textiles	--	0.5	--	0.6	20.0	0.9	50.0	0.6
Machine op - asst'd	8.8	2.9	12.3	4.2	19.7	2.9	--	0.9
Fabricators, assemblers, handworking	4.0	2.8	--	3.8	17.8	2.9	13.6	3.9
Clerical/Office								
Office clerical	3.2	11.4	10.7	7.8	8.8	10.1	25.1	7.1
Data entry	50.0	0.9	--	.8	6.7	0.9	38.9	0.6
Information clerk	4.8	1.7	--	3.1	7.6	3.7	14.3	2.1
Secretary/typist	1.9	11.2	--	7.3	4.0	11.4	18.2	3.7
Bookkeeping/related	6.2	7.7	--	2.8	10.7	7.5	--	0.9
Total % of all jobs		60.3		70.8		63.1		71.2

% impoverished corresponds to the percentage of women in that occupation are live at a level between poverty and twice poverty (see Table 1)

% all jobs refers to the percentage of all women's employment represented by that occupation in each racial and marital subgroup

Source: U.S. Department of Commerce (1983)

REPORTED ACCIDENTS, INJURIES AND ILLNESSES IN OCCUPATIONS OF THE WORKING POOR

We now turn from a consideration of which occupational groups are poverty-stricken or impoverished to a discussion of the work environment of the working poor. One measure of health and safety conditions in work environments is the number of injuries and illnesses reported to the workers' compensation agency in each state. It is widely recognized that workers' compensation data represent only a fraction of the true rate of disease and disability that occurs in the workplace (U.S. Department of Labor, 1980). Compensation data are largely reflective of severe, acute conditions such as those resulting from traumatic in-

Table 3b. Women in Selected Occupations Employed Full-Time
And Living in Impoverishment: Less than 45 Years of Age

Occupation	Married				Unmarried			
	White		Non-white		White		Non-white	
	% impover-ished	% all jobs	% impover-ished	% all jobs	% impover-ished	% all jobs	% impover-ished	% all jobs
Service								
Food services (prep)	5.4	1.1	3.8	3.0	7.5	1.3	17.2	3.0
Waitress/bartending	13.3	1.0	--	0.8	14.1	2.0	12.5	0.9
Personal services	15.0	1.1	20.0	1.1	45.5	0.8	69.3	1.3
Cosmetology/barber	18.0	1.0	25.8	0.5	27.8	1.2	27.3	1.1
Private household	40.5	0.1	75.0	0.5	40.0	0.1	83.3	1.2
Building services	26.4	0.7	25.0	2.7	46.0	1.3	68.1	3.3
Health Services	13.8	2.7	33.2	7.1	26.2	3.1	39.3	6.0
Retail Sales	11.3	3.6	27.6	3.0	21.0	4.0	44.6	4.5
Industry/Agriculture								
Agriculture/Forestry	33.4	1.2	75.0	0.5	29.6	0.7	30.6	0.5
Stitchers & Sewers	19.2	0.4	27.9	4.2	39.6	1.0	70.3	0.7
Laundry	20.0	1.8	61.5	0.8	42.9	0.2	85.7	2.8
Textiles	16.7	0.1	18.2	1.3	42.8	0.5	57.2	1.4
Machine op - asst'd	6.9	3.0	26.3	4.3	18.9	2.0	53.0	3.9
Fabricators,assemblers, handworking	7.1	2.4	21.4	2.8	31.7	2.4	33.1	3.8
Clerical/Office								
Office clerical	4.6	10.7	10.5	11.1	12.6	9.8	31.3	11.7
Data entry	--	1.2	1.7	2.5	11.1	1.3	21.5	1.9
Information clerk	4.9	3.9	6.0	3.8	21.1	3.4	31.9	4.8
Secretary/typist	3.9	14.4	10.2	12.2	16.8	14.3	31.0	10.2
Bookkeeping/related	4.6	6.6	10.5	2.2	21.3	5.4	44.4	3.2
Total % of all jobs		57.0		64.4		54.8		66.2

% impoverished corresponds to the percentage of women in that occupation
are live at a level between poverty and twice poverty (see Table 1)

% all jobs refers to the percentage of all women's employment represented
by that occupation in each racial and marital subgroup

Source: U.S. Department of Commerce (1983)

jury. Occupational diseases are virtually unrecorded in the system. Chronic effects of exposures to toxins or other hazards, such as the development of cancer, the occurrence of adverse reproductive outcomes (e.g., infertility, spontaneous abortions, birth defects, perinatal death and developmental defects), the onset of chronic obstructive lung diseases or other systemic afflictions, are not likely to be recorded either because of a failure to appropriately diagnose the occupational causation of the disease or because of bureaucratic barriers, such as limitations on time for reporting a disease, which effectively excludes most conditions with a long latency period between exposure and onset.

The data in Table 4 shows that entire sectors of the female population, such as private household workers, simply never make their way into the workers' compensation system or are excluded from the system by statute. There were only 118 claims filed by private household workers in the 27 participating states.

Despite its limitations, however, compensation data are one of the few sources of quantitative information on the extent of injuries and illnesses on the job. In this paper I have extracted data from the Bureau of Labor Statistics' Supplemental Data Set, described above, on the number of claims filed, the nature of the injury or illness and the part of the body affected for most of the major occupational categories in which full-time women employees were found to be living in impoverishment or poverty. Exact occupational matching at the detailed job level is not readily possible since the Bureau of Labor Statistics and the Census Bureau use different systems for classifying occupations. These data are presented in Tables 4, 5 and 6. The reader is, however, cautioned, once again, to regard them as a *conservative* estimate of the true rate of injury, and certainly of the true rate of systemic disease attributable in whole or in part to workplace factors.

There were 94,001 claims filed by women in the selected occupational groupings in 1980. Fifty-five percent of all claims are for sprains, strains, fractures, concussions and herniations, while lacerations, puncture wounds and abrasions represent another 24%. Infectious diseases, including hepatitis, represent 0.4% of the claims among all workers but 0.9% among health service workers. Four percent of the injuries are related to exposure to temperature extremes, primarily burns. Waitresses and food service workers have more than double and triple rates for these injuries, corresponding to 9.0% and 12.9% respectively, compared to all workers in the other occupations with impoverished or poverty-stricken workers.

Inflammation of the joints, including bursitis, tenosynovitis and other conditions affecting joints, tendons and muscles, but not including strains and sprains, represents 3.1% of the total reported injuries and illnesses. Sewing machine operators and factory workers, however, experience much higher rates, with 6.4% and 7.4% of their total claims attributable to these conditions. Among clerical workers, 1% of their total claims are also attributable to injury to the joints.

Tenosynovitis, inflammation of the muscle sheath in the wrist,

TABLE 4. NUMBERS AND PERCENTS OF INJURIES AND ILLNESSES REPORTED TO STATE WORKERS' COMPENSATION AGENCIES BY WOMEN IN LOW-PAYING OCCUPATIONS**
Type of Injury Reported***

Occupation	Amputation	Sprains/abrasions	Infections	Skin cond'ns	Burns/cold	Hearing	Joint disease	Poisoning	Radiations	Varicos-ities	Mental Disorders	Occup. Diseases	Unclass.	National Estimates##
Retail Sales	8(0.2)	3174(81.5)	5(0.1)	10(0.9)	48(1.2)	—	30(0.8)	29(.7)	1(0.0)	8(5.8)	28(0.7)	28(0.7)	528(13.6)	10,253
Factory Work	324(1.1)	22895(75.3)	24(0.1)	503(1.7)	618(2.0)	34(0.1)	225(7.4)	320(1.1)	14(0.0)	37(0.1)	48(0.2)	915(3.0)	2408(7.9)	79,995
Laundry	3(1.1)	783(76.6)	3(0.2)	18(1.7)	56(5.5)	—	21(2.1)	10(0.9)	—	3(0.3)	3(0.3)	17(1.7)	100(9.8)	2,671
Sewers/Stitchers	10(.4)	1891(76.3)	2(0.1)	55(2.1)	102(3.9)	—	16(6.4)	22(0.8)	—	3(0.1)	1(0.0)	47(1.8)	209(8.1)	6,837
Textile	8(3.3)	181(74.0)	—	5(2.0)	2(1.0)	—	14(5.9)	1(0.4)	—	—	—	5(2.0)	28(11.5)	642
Farm	7(0.5)	937(73.4)	3(0.2)	36(2.8)	17(1.3)	1(0.1)	23(1.8)	27(2.1)	2(0.0)	1(0.1)	1(0.1)	21(1.6)	204(15.9)	3,363
Building Services	6(0.1)	6093(81.7)	12(0.1)	94(1.3)	165(2.2)	—	111(1.5)	97(1.3)	2(0.0)	19(0.3)	20(0.3)	81(1.1)	767(10.3)	19,647
Food Services	93(0.7)	1115(74.5)	15(0.1)	139(1.0)	821(12.9)	—	123(0.9)	62(0.4)	1(0.0)	25(0.2)	17(0.1)	119(0.8)	1209(8.5)	37,258
Waitress/Bar	11(0.2)	4207(76.4)	7(0.2)	28(0.5)	495(9.0)	1(0.0)	54(1.0)	17(0.3)	1(0.0)	5(0.1)	5(0.1)	45(0.8)	633(11.5)	14,489
Personal Services	5(0.1)	3261(76.1)	30(0.6)	47(1.1)	222(5.2)	20(0.5)	41(1.0)	47(1.1)	1(0.0)	8(0.2)	16(0.4)	35(0.8)	553(12.9)	11,274
Cosmetologists/Barbers	—	206(58.8)	2(0.4)	50(14.3)	12(3.4)	—	15(4.4)	10(2.7)	—	—	2(0.6)	18(5.0)	37(10.6)	926
Health Services	20(0.1)	19832(87.4)	214(0.9)	166(0.7)	197(0.9)	3(0.0)	104(0.5)	84(0.4)	1(0.0)	20(0.1)	41(0.2)	138(0.6)	1869(8.2)	59,708
Housework	1(0.8)	96(81.3)	—	2(1.3)	3(2.1)	—	1(0.4)	3(2.1)	—	—	1(0.4)	2(1.3)	12(10.2)	311
Clerical	2(0.3)	411(75.5)	1(0.1)	3(0.5)	3(0.6)	—	6(1.0)	7(1.3)	—	1(0.2)	22(3.9)	6(1.0)	22(3.9)	1,439
Totals	497(.5)	74593(78.9)	253(.4)	1155(1.2)	3761(4.0)	57(.1)	2966(3.1)	733(.8)	21(0)	130(.1)	204(.2)	1477(1.6)	8642(3.4)	/248,813

*Based on the U.S. Bureau of Labor Statistics Supplementary Data System Microdata Files, 1980

** This is a recoding into broad Illness/Injury categories by the author. Original categories available upon request.

##Estimate by the author is based on relative population of women in the 27 States to the population of the United States, applying statistical weights in data and other injuries to the joints are associated with rapid, repetitive motions, particularly if carried out in an awkward position, such as with the wrist flexed rather than straight. The 7.4% of total claim rate among factory workers is reflective of the jobs that most women factory workers hold: assembling of small parts and small machines. Many of these jobs require continual hand motion, often with a simultaneous flexing of the wrist, such as in tightening of screws or packaging of products on the assembly line. In Table 5 we can see that in this group 9.5% of the claims are for injury to the wrist, although some of these wrist injuries may not be to the joints but rather to the bones.

Among cosmetologists and barbers, dermatitis represents 14% of the claims, while skin diseases are 1.2% of the total claims. This is reflective of the dermatological risks (both of irritation

TABLE 5. BODY-PART AFFECTED BY INJURIES REPORTED TO STATE WORKERS' COMPENSATION AGENCIES BY WOMEN IN LOW-PAYING OCCUPATIONS*
(Percent distribution)

Occupation	Head/Neck	Arms	Wrist	Hands	Trunk	Back	Legs	Multiple Systems	Systemic
Retail Sales	7.2	3.4	4.1	13.2	8.0	23.9	24.5	12.5	3.2
Factory Work	6.0	7.2	9.5	27.5	8.9	19.1	12.1	6.7	2.9
Laundry	5.3	6.1	5.7	15.2	11.9	30.0	15.0	7.2	3.5
Sewers/Stitchers	5.9	6.3	9.4	35.4	7.4	18.5	7.9	6.5	2.8
Textile	2.9	7.6	9.8	27.8	11.1	22.3	9.8	7.0	1.6
Farm	7.6	5.2	5.3	14.6	12.1	19.6	21.3	9.4	5.0
Building Service	6.0	5.0	4.4	11.0	11.2	28.6	20.7	9.5	3.6
Food Services	4.6	6.4	4.5	30.7	7.3	18.2	17.5	8.4	2.4
Waitress/Bar	4.9	5.4	4.4	18.0	8.7	19.6	26.1	10.7	2.2
Personal Services	11.6	3.6	3.6	8.9	9.7	26.5	20.9	11.5	3.9
Cosmetologists/ Barbers	5.6	5.0	8.1	37.5	5.8	9.1	13.6	9.4	5.8
Health Services	5.2	3.4	3.4	6.7	12.8	44.5	11.8	9.5	2.7
Housework	3.8	6.2	7.2	6.8	10.6	24.6	24.5	12.3	3.8
Clerical	7.2	4.0	3.9	10.9	9.0	22.8	23.5	10.6	8.1
Total	5.8%	5.5%	6.0%	19.6%	9.8%	26.5%	15.3%	8.6%	2.9%

*Based on the U.S. Bureau of Labor Statistics Supplementary Data System Microdata Files, 1980

and allergy) associated with frequent wetting of the hands and contact with hairdressing and coloring agents.

The Supplemental Data System also classifies claims as to the body part affected. These data have been extracted and analyzed by the occupations under consideration here and are presented in Table 5. Once again, despite the underreporting, the distribution of claims by body part provide insight into the major occupational injury hazards. Injuries to the back are the most prevalent, accounting for almost half of the claims filed by health services and one-third of those in laundry work. Of all total claims 26.5% involve injury to the back.

Women appear to be at particular risk for injuries to the hands, and in some occupations, like sewing and stitching, hand injuries account for more than one-third of all claims. It is interesting to note that injuries to the legs among women in retail sales have a prevalence rate almost twice that of all women in this group. This can logically be attributed to the long hours of standing required by most retail-sales jobs. Unfortunately, no independent studies have been published on this question of the relationship between occupations that involve long periods of standing and the development of such dysfunctions as varicosities.

Despite the limitations in total reporting to the system, and the obvious absence of data on occupational diseases, analysis of the relative incidence of acute conditions within occupational groups compared to the incidence among the group as a whole does provide some insight into occupation-specific hazards. Further, we gain insight into the minimum total burden of injury across the United States. The claims in the Supplemental Data System are accorded a statistical weight in order to permit extrapolation to national rates. In 1980, female employees in the 27 states in the data set represented 38% of the total number of female employees in the United States, according to the 1980 Census. The last column in Table 4 gives the estimated national injury rate of 248,805 when extrapolated from the percentage representation using the SDS weights.

Analysis of workers' compensation data shows that despite the obvious underreporting by women in several major occupations, and, despite the almost virtual absence of data on occupational disease, as well as the other impediments to accurate recording of illness that exist, a quarter of a million full-time female workers holding jobs in occupations employing significant numbers of impoverished or poverty-stricken workers are seriously enough injured or disabled on the job to file a claim in their state workers' compensation system, using the extrapolated figures.

OCCUPATIONAL HAZARDS AND DISEASES OF POOR WORKING WOMEN

Occupational health problems of women workers have not been well-defined nor sufficiently studied (Hunt, 1982). A review of the occupational hazards that poor working women face may require assumptions and extrapolations of medical and scientific data on hazards and effects in other occupations or in experimental settings. In this section I will present a brief review of chemical hazards primarily associated with cancer, adverse reproductive outcomes, occupational lung diseases and skin effects among women employed in the most impoverished sectors, together with information on safety hazards and stress. These data are summarized in Table 6.

Stellman and Stellman (1981) have reviewed the major female-dominated occupations in which known carcinogens were present. These include some sterilizing agents like ethylene oxide and ultraviolet light, vinyl chloride and various dyes used in the cosmetology and textile industries. Since the time of that review, new scientific research has found increased human risks for cancer from formaldehyde and strong experimental evidence of carcinogenicity for methylene chloride, now known to be a carcinogen. These two chemicals are widely used solvents in these professions (Women's Occupational Health Resource Center News, 1986; Dept. Health and Human Services, 1986). In fact, the Food and Drug Administration, in proposing a ban on the use of methylene chloride as a propellant, has estimated the risk for lung cancer to be between 1 in 100 and 1 in 1000 among cosmetologists who work with the substance on a full-time basis. Women in the microelectronics industry and in other factory work are also commonly exposed to this highly volatile solvent but no estimates of their relative risks are currently available.

Agricultural workers, a particularly impoverished sector

Table 6. Potential Occupational Health Hazards in Selected Occupations Characterized By Impoverishment and Poverty of Significant Fractions Full-Time Female Workers

Occupation	Known or Suspected Cancer Hazard*	Other Hazards
Health services	Sterilizing Agents and Disinfectants	Electrical shocks
nurses' aides	(ethylene oxide, formaldehyde,	Slips and falls (wet floors)
orderlies	ultraviolet light)	Back injuries (handling patients)
practical nurses	Hepatitis B	Skin irritation (wet hands; allergy to
cleaners	Radioisotopes	drugs)
	Cancer drugs	Puncture wounds/lacerations from needles
	Ionizing Radiation	sharp objects
		Shiftwork
		Infectious Agents
Clothing and Textile	Benzidine-type dyes	Noise from machines and looms
workers	Asbestos	Cotton dust ("Brown lung")
	Formaldehyde	Eye and hand injuries (needles)
	BCME (from permanent press finishes)	Ergonomic stressors (wrist/back)
	Tris (flame retardants)	Pulmonary irritants (dyes, additives)
		Stress (assembly line and piecework)
Laundry Workers	Contaminant dusts (asbestos,	High temperature and humidity
	beryllium)	Enzyme detergents (lung sensitivity)
	Dry cleaning solvents (TCE,	Ergonomic stressors (lifting and carrying
	perchloroethylene)	laundry)
		Noise from machines
		Standing
hairdressers and	Hair dyes	Standing
cosmetologists	Asbestos from dryers	Puncture wounds (hair)
	Ultraviolet light	Dermatitis (allergic and irritation)
	Solvents	
	Formaldehyde (preservative)	
	Propellants (methylene chloride	
	and formerly vinyl chloride)	
Agricultural workers	Organochlorine pesticides:	Ergonomic stressors (bending,
	aldrin/dieldrin, endrin, Kepone,	stretching and carrying)
	methoxychlor, Mirex, DDT, lindane,	Poor personal hygiene facilities
	chlordane/heptachlor, toxaphene	Hot temperatures
	Arsenic pesticide and herbicides	Machine injuries
	Phenoxy herbicides: 2,4-D and 2,4,5-T	
Assembly workers;	Methylene chloride	Timed, repetitive piecework
Solders;	Polychlorinated biphenyls (PCBs)	Ergonomic stresses (rapid, repetitive
Microelectronics	Nitrosamines (in cutting oils)	motions)
	Cadmium and other metals	Shiftwork
Household Workers;	Cleaners may contain methylene	Isolation on the job
Building Services	chloride; nitrosamines in furniture	Infectious agents
	polish	Dermatitis from irritating substances
		Safety hazards
		Poor job security
Food Service		Temperature extremes
		Ergonomic stresses
		Dermatitis from allergens in food and
		wet hands
		Infectious agents (customers' leftovers)
		Noisy machines
Waitress/bartenders	Cigarette smoke	Standing and carrying
		Noise
		Infectious agents

* Many of the entries in this table are adapted from Stellman and Stellman (1983). Other entries are taken from sources given in references.

among full-time employed workers, are exposed to a wide variety of pesticides and herbicides, many of which are carcinogenic. No major epidemiologic study of the long-term consequences of these exposures has been done. Similarly, laundry workers can be exposed to toxic dusts that contaminate clothing and can be liberated during the handling for laundering. Beryllium and silica are known contaminants for laundry workers (Cohen & Positano, 1986; Evans & Posner, 1971). Again, however, no studies of long-term risks are available, although Li and co-workers have reported cases of asbestos-associated cancer in women whose only exposure to asbestos was the laundering of their husband's work clothing (Li et al., 1978). More mundane risks, such as lacerations and puncture wounds from sharp objects, can also be a serious problem, particularly among health service workers whose risk for infections like hepatitis B are thus seriously increased.

Health service workers, such as aides and orderlies or janitorial workers, can be exposed to carcinogenic sterilizing agents, as well as to hepatitis B virus, which is a risk factor for primary liver cancer. They may be exposed to antineoplastic drugs (cancer drugs), which can contaminate work surfaces, and to cancer patient wastes (Stellman & Zoloth, 1986). Many of these drugs are potent carcinogens and may also present other serious systemic occupational hazards, such as reproductive risks. Many health services workers are also laundry and food service workers and so share the risks of these occupations.

The hazards of housework to household workers are not well-documented either. Rosenberg (1984) has reviewed the hazards of household chemicals and compiled a list of at least twelve groups of common household products that can cause serious local effects on the skin or the eyes or can lead either to chronic or acute systemic poisoning. She based her work on information from consumer protection agencies, as well as from occupational and environmental health advocacy groups. No major studies of the health of household workers are available. It should also be noted that National Safety Council statistics on accidents have always found the home to be a greater source of injury than the workplace. Since the home *is* the workplace of the household worker, it is not unreasonable to propose that the household worker is at serious risk for accidental injury on the job.

Dusts are another type of occupational hazard affecting the working poor. Byssinosis, or "Brown Lung," is a chronic irreversible lung disease associated with inhalation of cotton dust, irrespective of whether the worker smokes (Bouhuys, 1986). Other organic dusts that can produce an allergic or other serious reaction and are of particular significance to women have been reviewed by Stellman and Stellman (1983). The list of agents or afflictions includes:

- farmers' lung (moldy hay);
- mushroom workers' lung (mushroom compost);
- bird fanciers' lung (pigeon, parrot and other droppings);
- chicken raisers' disease;
- extrinsic allergic alveolitis from contaminated humidifiers, air conditioners, heating systems;
- attacks from "housedusts" (probably attributable to dust mite *Dermatophagoides sp.*).

As we have seen in the analysis of the injuries and illnesses recorded in the workers' compensation system, the hands and wrists of female workers are a major site of insult, and tenosynovitis has already been mentioned as one problem. Allergic skin reactions (contact dermatitis) and dermatitis arising from continual exposure to wet conditions and/or irritating substances, can also injure the hands. Some of the chemicals associated with dermatological effects are provided in Table 6 as well.

Reproductive hazards that have been associated with outcomes such as infertility, spontaneous abortions and miscarriage can be found in the working environments of many of the working poor (Hatch, 1984; Polis, 1986), although very little human evidence is available that permits us to quantify the risks encountered. Some infectious agents are known reproductive hazards and it is well-established that women working in child-care facilities, health-care services and other personal services are at increased risk for occupationally caused infectious diseases, although the magnitude of the relative risks they suffer is not well-defined (Polis, 1986; Hunt, 1979). Many carcinogenic agents are also reproductive hazards as well, but insufficient data are available to provide a comprehensive list.

Physical hazards are also found in the workplace environment of the working poor. High levels of noise from machinery and looms characterize laundry work and textile work, and many textile factories operate at or near the maximum average noise level permitted by OSHA. The safety hazards in these jobs include electrical shock, falls and sprains. These unsafe conditions are the ones primarily reflected in the workers' compensation data reviewed above.

Finally, it is now widely recognized that occupational stress is a major risk factor for a large number of diseases and dysfunctions. Physical and chemical hazards and organizational factors, as well as the absence of sufficient money to provide for daily necessities and for amenities to help women cope with their multiple roles while employed full-time outside the home, may have serious adverse health effects the working poor. Recent work by Muller (1986a, 1986b) has shown that women in the lowest occupational categories and with multiple-role obligations suffer from the poorest health and lowest levels of satisfaction and life happiness.

CONCLUSIONS AND RECOMMENDATIONS

One can conclude from the review of the literature and from the data on injuries and illnesses that being employed full-time, yet impoverished or living in frank poverty, is not good for one's health. The working poor are at risk for ill-health from bad working conditions, from high stress levels and from insufficient means to do anything about it or to provide assistance for themselves.

This analysis of data on the economic well-being of women workers from the U.S. Census and on the occupational health and well-being from state workers' compensation boards clearly shows that a large number of American women are both impoverished and at-risk for developing occupationally related maladies and injuries. It is also clear that an insufficient data base is available for fully delineating the identity and extent of risk factors present and the actual level of ill-health and injury that is occurring. Urgent attention is needed in the area of improving hazard recognition, diagnosing illnesses and injuries, and reporting them to compensation agencies and to the medical and scientific communities.

Despite the dearth of exact information on risks and adverse effects, the large numbers of injuries that are already occurring indicate the presence of agents capable of inducing grave health effects in the workplaces of the working poor, and clearly demonstrate the need for immediate development of prevention programs to eliminate occupational injuries and diseases. Unlike with many other chronic diseases where no cause is apparent or controllable, occupational diseases are artificially created and can, in general, be eliminated through appropriate workplace design or other control mechanisms. Such control is of the utmost necessity and urgency.

Women's occupations, and in general, occupations of the working poor, are covered by few standards for exposures to toxins or other dangerous conditions. Some occupations, such as household work, may not be covered by workplace laws or standards at all. It is of urgent need to increase the regulatory attention given to these jobs both from a standards-setting and from an enforcement perspective. Too often a scale is constructed that rates high-injury industries such as construction and lumbering above traditionally female-dominated work and hence effectively eliminates female-dominated occupations from routine inspection or standards-making. These priority systems must be reexamined and reestablished to eliminate their inherent biases against working women.

REFERENCES

Bouhuys, A., Schoenber, J.B., Beck, G.J. et al. (1986),"Epidemiology of chronic lung disease in a cotton mill community," Lung 154, 167-186.

Brandeis, Elizabeth in John R. Commons et al. (1918) "History of Labor in the U.S. Volume 1. New York: Macmillan, p. 462.

Chavkin, Wendy, ed. (1984), "Double Exposure: Women's Health Hazards on the Job and At Home," New York: Monthly Review Press.

Cohen, Beverly S. and Rock Positano (1986), "Resuspension of Dust from Work Clothing as a Source of Inhalation Exposure," Am Ind. Hyg Assoc J (47), 255-258.

Evans, D.J. and E. Posner (1971), "Pneumoconiosis in laundry workers," Environ. Res (4), 121-128.

Hatch, Maureen (1984). "Mother, Father, Worker: Men and Women and the Reproduction Risks of Work," pp. 161-180, in Chavkin, op cit.

Hunt, Vilma R. (no date), "Occupational Health Problems of Pregnant Women: A Report and Recommendations for the Office of the Secretary, DHEW," Order No. SA-5304-75.

Hunt, Vilma (1979), Work and the Health of Women. Boca Raton: CRC press.

Hunt, Vilma R. (1982), "Health of Women at Work," Chicago: Northwestern University program on Women.

Li, F.B., J. Lokich and J. Lapey et al. (1978), "Familial mesothelium after intense asbestos exposure at their home," JAMA 240(5): 467. *Muller* v. *Oregon,* 208 U.S. 412 (1908).

Muller, Charlotte (1986a). "Health and Health Care of Employed Women and Homemakers: Family Factors," Women and Health 11(1),7-26.

Muller, Charlotte (1986b). "Health and Health Care of Employed Adults: Occupation and Gender," Women and Health 11(1), 27-47.

Polis, Michael et al. (1986) Transmission of Giardia lamblia from a day care center to the community, AJPHA 76(9), 1142-1144. Ratner, Ronnie Steinberg (1980). "The Paradox of Protection: Maximum hours legislation in the United States," Int'l Labour Review,185-198.

Rosenberg, Harriet G. (1984), "The Home is the Workplace: Hazards, Stress and Pollutants in the Household," p. 219-245 in Chavkin, W., op cit.

Stellman, Jeanne Mager (1977), "Women's Work, Women's Health: Myths and Realities" New York: Pantheon.

Stellman, Steven D. and Jeanne M. Stellman (1981), "Women's Occupations, Smoking and Cancer and Other Diseases," CA 11(1), 29-43.

Stellman, Jeanne M. and Steven D. Stellman (1983). "Occupational Lung Disease and Cancer Risk in Women," Occupational Health Nursing, 40-46, November.

Stellman, Jeanne M. and Stephen Zoloth (1986). "Cancer Chemotherapeutic as Occupational Hazards: A Literature Review," Cancer Investigation 4(2), 127-135.

U.S. Department of Commerce, Bureau of the Census (1983), "Census of Population and Housing: 1980 Public-Use Microdata Samples," Washington.

U.S. Dept. Health and Human Services, Food and Drug Administration (1986), "Cosmetics; Proposed Ban on the Use of Methylene Chloride as an Ingredient of Aerosol Cosmetic Products," Federal Register, 21 CFR Part 700, 51551-51559.

U.S. Department of Labor, Assistant Secretary for Policy (1980), Evaluation and Research, "An Interim Report to Congress on Occupational Disease," Submitted to Congress, June 1980. U.S. Department of Labor, Bureau of Labor Statistics (1982). "Supplemental Data Systems, Microdata Files, 1980 Edition," Washington D.C.

Women's Occupational Health Resource Center News (1986), Volume 7 No (5), Brooklyn: Foundation for Worker, Veteran and Environmental Health Inc., for reviews of recent studies.

Illness-Engendered Poverty
Among the Elderly

Lois Grau, RN, PhD

SUMMARY. This paper presents an overview of the economic situation of elderly women in the United States. Its focus is on "illness-engendered poverty," a type of poverty that results from the inadequacies of Medicare coverage of long-term care and the subsequent need of many elderly to "spend down" into poverty in order to qualify for means-tested, publicly financed health and social programs. The consequences of Medicaid eligibility requirements and system incentives on the economic and social well-being of older women and their families are discussed.

The decade of the 1960s was characterized by a societal sensitivity to the plight of the disadvantaged—minority groups, women, and the aged. Aged Americans were portrayed as disenfranchised citizens, abandoned by their families and vulnerable to the ravages of illness and poverty. Social concern for their plight was reflected in the development of special interest and advocacy groups for the elderly, and legislative actions such as Medicare, Medicaid, and the Older American's Act—programs designed to enhance the quality of life of aged Americans.

The situation is different in the 1980s. Rather than asking what society can do for the aged, policymakers are questioning whether, in fact, we have not done too much for older Americans (Kutza, 1981). Current interest revolves around issues of intergenerational transfers and responsibilities, family care of elderly members, and categorical entitlements to costly old age programs. This conservative shift in perspective can be ex-

Lois Grau is Associate Director, Brookdale Research Institute on Aging, Third Age Center, Fordham University, 113 W. 60th Street, New York, NY 10023.

103

plained, at least in part, by two sets of factors: the reorientation of political interest from the "war against poverty" to issues of national defense and the federal budget deficit; and data that indicate that today's elderly are far better off economically than their counterparts of twenty years ago.

Today's elderly *are* economically better off than their predecessors. For the first time in recent history, the proportion of older people as a whole who fall below the poverty line, 13 percent, is smaller than that for the population as a whole (Uhlenberg & Salmon, 1986). This statistic, however, fails to capture the economic diversity of the elderly population where a significant minority of persons enter old age with incomes near the poverty line and become impoverished during the course of aging. Traditional economic measures do not reflect the dynamics of poverty, particularly the interplay between poverty and illness among older Americans. Those who enter old age in poverty are more likely to suffer poorer health than their more affluent counterparts, and chronic illness among the more affluent can lead to impoverishment as a result of public policies that require individuals to "spend down" to poverty levels in order to qualify for publicly supported health and social programs.

In addition, while it has been suggested that the elderly poor are better off than those with higher incomes because of their entitlement to publicly supported health and social service programs, the poor still receive significantly less care relative to the rest of the population, despite their dramatic increase in health service utilization since the advent of Medicaid (Davis, Gold, & Makuc, 1981). As will be described later, Medicaid-financed services are often inadequate to meet the multiple health and social needs of the elderly who wish to remain in the community during the last years of their lives. This problem is particularly acute for those who live alone, the vast majority of whom are women.

WHO ARE THE ELDERLY POOR?

Today, the majority of older Americans are doing comparatively well. Their relative health has improved consistently and substantially over the past two decades (Palmore, 1986) as has their economic well-being. Also, earlier myths which portrayed the aged as socially isolated and abandoned by their children have been disproven. Most older persons remain in regular and frequent contact with their children. Family and friends provide what Cantor (1983) terms a "social care system" in which continuous or intermittent ties and interchanges of assistance help older persons to maintain their psychological, social and physical integrity over time. Only when this system breaks down, or the need for care and assistance exceeds available resources, do elderly persons turn to formal health and social services and face the question of how to pay for needed care.

But what is true for most is not true for all. Currently 13 percent of the elderly live below the poverty line. A significant number of others, while not poor in terms of national poverty income standards, find it difficult or impossible to meet high living costs or purchase needed medical, health or social services. Those most vulnerable are the "near poor," with incomes that fall just above the poverty line. Currently, more elderly fall into this category than any other age group (Lehrman, 1980).

Moreover, poverty among the elderly is not a random event — its mostly likely victims are women. Although older women are economically better off in absolute terms than their counterparts of earlier decades, one out of five lives in poverty today. Women comprise 60 percent of the elderly but make up 72 percent of the aged poor. Older women as a whole have lower average incomes than older men. In 1985 the average monthly Social Security benefit for women was $399 as compared to $521 for men (U.S. Department of Health and Human Services, 1985).

Women are also at a disadvantage because of their minimal participation in job-related pension plans. Only 20 percent of aged women receive pension benefits as compared to 43 percent of aged men. Women who do qualify for benefits receive only one-half the pension income of men. Nor have women been as able as men to upgrade their economic status through participation in the labor force after retirement. In 1984, only 7 percent of women as compared with 17 percent of men over the age of 65 were employed (Congressional Clearinghouse on the Future, 1985).

Unmarried women are the most likely to be poor. Twenty-two

percent of all widows are poor, a poverty rate one and one-half times that of the aged population as a whole (U.S. Bureau of the Census, 1985). Older women are three times as likely as older men to be unmarried and thus rely on a single income. This is the result of men's propensity to marry younger women and the greater longevity of women. Also, single women generally receive lower Social Security payments because of lower preretirement incomes and their tendency to engage in work not recognized by the Social Security system, such as child care and the care of aged family members.

Minority membership increases the risk of poverty in old age. Blacks and Hispanics represent the poorest groups of aged Americans. Thirty-six percent of aged Blacks and 38 percent of aged Hispanics lived in extreme poverty in 1982 (U.S. Congress, 1983). In 1981, minority women fared even worse, with 80 percent of aged Black women (Women's Equity Action League, 1985) and 50 percent of older Hispanic women in poverty (Berger, 1983) compared to 20 percent of all aged women.

POVERTY AND ILLNESS

Those who are poor and old are also more likely to suffer from ill health. Women and minorities with low incomes and low educational levels have a higher incidence of disease than their economically more affluent counterparts (Butler & Newacheck, 1981). Disease affects an individual's ability to carry out the routine activities of daily living, behaviors that are most important in terms of physical, social, and psychological well-being. Again, such functional-impairment rates are disproportionately high among the poor, the majority of whom are women and who are most vulnerable, with rates twice as high as those of the nonpoor aged (U.S. Department of Health, Education, and Welfare, 1983).

Older women live longer than older men, and they are more likely than men to experience multiple, chronic, and increasingly debilitating diseases prior to death. Men are more likely to die of shorter-term fatal illnesses. Thus, many poor older women must contend with their own health deficits and those of their spouses.

The burden of caretaking, the personal losses of widowhood, and often their own ill-health are usually accompanied by few resources beyond those available from family, friends and public programs.

ILLNESS AND POVERTY

Cross-sectional economic data on poverty among the elderly fail to capture the dynamics of the process of impoverishment over time. The importance of this problem is highlighted by recent work underscoring the fluidity of poverty throughout the life span, where many persons, including the elderly, move in and out of poverty as a result of situational factors that elevate or deplete expendable income (Holden, Burkhauser & Myers, 1986).

Age-related situational factors increase the risk of impoverishment. Widowhood is possibly the most economically devastating event of this kind. In addition, both older men and women also typically experience a reduction in income after retirement. This relative impoverishment may be balanced for some persons by age-related economic advantages—lower living expenses, such as less need for clothing and transportation due to the exit from the work force, no responsibility for minor-age children, age-related tax advantages, and programs such as Medicare and Medicaid. However, aging is associated with certain economic disadvantages and deficits such as fixed incomes in an inflationary economy, age-related job discrimination for those who wish to work, and the high cost of health care not covered by Medicare. The interplay of the assets and deficits for aged persons is largely dependent on personal expectations, total economic assets, health status, and ability to rely on support from family members.

Of particular interest here is illness-engendered poverty, which occurs when health-care costs exceed an individual's ability to pay. Those most likely to fall on the deficit side of the old-age economic equation as a result of illness are persons whom Smeeding (1986) refers to as the " 'tweeners," individuals in the lower-middle income range who are without benefit of Medigap supplemental health insurance and in-kind housing subsidies and who rely on Social Security as their primary source of cash income. When faced with illness, 'tweeners are likely to have no choice but to spend down to penury in order to qualify for means-tested cash and in-kind transfers in the form of Medicaid and Supplemental Security Income. Among middle-income elderly, three in five meet two of the three conservative inclusion criteria for 'tweeners. As might be expected, single elderly women are particularly vulnerable. Two-thirds of middle-income, single women aged 65 to 74 who live alone are 'tweeners. This statistic increases to 76 percent for middle-income women aged 75 years or older.

Medicare and Medicaid

Medicare and Medicaid are the two major programs that pay for care for the elderly. Medicare is a health insurance program covering a substantial portion of the costs of hospital and physician services for individuals aged 65 and over, for certain disabled persons under age 65, and for persons with end-stage renal disease. It was designed to assist the elderly to obtain acute medical care services rather than long-term homecare or institutional care.

Much care and assistance that the elderly are most likely to require — dentures, hearing aids, and community or institutional long-term care — are not covered by the program. Medicare does not cover health prevention and promotion interventions for diseases most likely to afflict older women such as breast cancer, osteoporosis, and diabetes. These failures of the program necessitate high out-of-pocket expenditures and, for some, eventual reliance on welfare. In 1984, Medicare expended 63 billion dollars on hospital services and one-quarter billion dollars on physician services. In that same year, less than 1 percent of total Medicare expenditures was devoted to home care and only 3.1 percent to nursing-home care (U.S. Congress, 1985). The costs of long-term care are not covered by private insurance either, which covers less than 1 percent of the nation's nursing-home bill (U.S. Department of Health and Human Services, 1984), and even less of the total costs of long-term home health care.

Medicare expenditures, although escalating rapidly, still pay only 45 percent of the total cost of health care services for the nation's elderly. Elderly persons with incomes below $10,000 (in 1984 dollars) spend roughly 16.5 percent of their income on direct health care costs or health insurance, while those with incomes under $5,000 expend 21 percent of their total income for these purposes. In 1961, prior to the implementation of Medicare, this figure was only 11 percent, even at poverty-line incomes (Smeeding, 1986). The poor, the majority of whom are women, bear a disproportionate share of this cost-sharing burden (Davis, 1986).

The majority of the poor and near-poor are not covered by supplemental "Medigap" insurance and thus face possible destitution should they experience a catastrophic illness. Supposedly, the Medicaid program covers persons unable to pay for needed health care not reimbursed by Medicare. Medicaid is a federal welfare program designed to provide medical care to the poor of all ages. Although participating states are required under federal guidelines to provide a minimal set of services, states have wide discretionary power over eligibility criteria, access, and utilization of funded services, leading to wide variation in expenditures among states (Harrington, Estes, Lee & Newcomer, 1986).

In most states, Medicaid eligibility is determined by complex formulas sufficiently strict that almost one-half of the nation's poor do not qualify for the program. Often Medicaid eligibility is tied to eligibility for other welfare benefits such as, in the case of the elderly, to Supplemental Security Income (Joe, Meltzer & Yu, 1985). As a result, individuals who thus qualify for Medicaid-supported services may have welfare incomes inadequate to support their continued residence in the community. This means that these individuals may have no choice but to accept nursing-home placement because of inadequate expendable income and limited Medicaid-supported community-based care. There are exceptions to these circumstances. A New York State long-term health care program is providing needed care in the home as long as costs do not exceed 75 percent of the Medicaid nursing-home reimbursement rate. However, the majority of states have yet to implement such important programs.

A related and serious problem are the economic consequences

of "spending down" on spouses, which disproportionately affect women. Medicaid policies require that spouses be economically responsible for each other. In New York State, for example, a women whose husband qualifies for Medicaid can retain no more than $8,900 of their joint life savings, and her monthly income cannot exceed Medicaid monthly income standards (Nickman, 1986). This impoverishment requirement virtually assures the wife's eventual inclusion on the Medicaid rolls should she become ill.

Medicaid currently pays roughly 48 percent of the nation's nursing-home bill. However, approximately 65 percent of the nation's nursing-home residents are on the Medicaid rolls. The difference between the two figures reflects the proportionally higher costs paid by private-pay residents, an unknown number of whom are at any one point in time in the process of spending down themselves. And for every married Medicaid nursing-home resident there is, somewhere, an impoverished spouse. (The exception is families who have divested assets.)

SPENDING DOWN: THREE CASE EXAMPLES

The process of spending down to Medicaid eligibility levels is, in and of itself, relatively simple — a matter of depleting economic assets on health care until eligibility levels are reached. Persons at lowest risk of spending down into illness-engendered poverty are typically those who are in good health or whose illness requires only periodic, short-term acute medical care; have Medigap insurance or the economic resources to cover Medicare co-payments; and have family on whom they can rely for personal care and household assistance; or, lastly, are able and willing to spend $2,400 to $5,000 per month on homecare or nursing-home care. Persons at greatest risk of illness-engendered poverty are those who have more or less the opposite characteristics — persons who suffer from chronic debilitating illness, who are of moderate income, and who lack needed informal support from family members.

The following cases demonstrate the complexities of "spending down" and the critical role that knowledge of the system plays in predicting spend-down outcomes. State-to-state variation in eligibility criteria and confusion about the economic consequences of spending down on family members (even among professionals who administer the system) are barriers to the education of the at-risk public.

The first case demonstrates the dilemma of a daughter who is economically dependent upon her ailing mother.

Case 1 — The Decision Not to Spend Down

Belle, and her only daughter Marilyn, aged 72, shared the expenses of a modest apartment. By pooling their incomes they were just able to make ends meet.

Belle died last spring at age 97. The real problems began seven months prior to her death when she sustained a fall and was hospitalized. Although no bones were broken, Belle became incontinent, bedridden, and confused in the hospital. Despite Belle's deterioration, Marilyn was informed that Belle would be discharged after seven days because hospitalization was no longer deemed medically necessary. Marilyn was given the choice of taking Belle home or placing her in the one local nursing home that would accept residents who would shortly qualify for Medicaid.

Marilyn faced a dilemma. She knew she could not adequately cope with Belle's personal care needs because she, herself, suffered from an eye disease and was physically weak as a result of a recently healed broken ankle. On the other hand, Marilyn found the nursing home to be a smelly and unpleasant place with staff who seemed to care little about Belle's problems. Moreover, should she institutionalize Belle, Marilyn would lose Belle's income, which she needed to help pay the rent. As a result, Marilyn felt she had no choice but to take Belle home.

Marilyn's life was thus reduced to caring for Belle and attempting to cope with Belle's confusion and constant demands. Medicare paid for an occasional visit from a Visiting Nurse and for a nurse's aide four hours a week, which helped, but did not relieve the sleepless nights or Marilyn's growing frustration and depression. One afternoon, after

Belle had yelled the same set of questions and insults at Marilyn for hours, Marilyn escaped outside and sat in the car for a few moments of peace and quiet. Soon, however, Belle somehow managed to unlock the back door and find Marilyn. Marilyn's frustration was such that she simply drove away, leaving Belle leaning on her walker in the driveway.

Belle died at home four months later. Today, Marilyn looks back with guilt at her occasional failures to cope with Belle's demands and to provide the constant love and care she believed her mother deserved. However, the interest on Belle's small estate of $18,000 has enabled Marilyn to continue, albeit just barely, to make ends meet.

The second case exemplifies the growing phenomenon of divestment of personal assets to reduce the state's "take" during the spend-down process, while the third case demonstrates the ignorance many Americans have about the eventual consequences of spending down.

Case 2 — "Gaming the System"

Peter did his homework. When his mother began to evidence frailty at age 80 he consulted legal experts in order to develop a strategy to protect at least some of her assets should she eventually require nursing-home care. He learned that if he divested her money two or more years prior to Medicaid application, these monies could not be recovered by the state.

Peter transferred all but $30,000 of his mother's assets to his name. $30,000 was retained in order to "buy in" to a high-quality nursing home should this become necessary, as local nursing homes of high repute gave admission preference to persons who could afford to pay out-of-pocket, i.e., spend down, for at least one year prior to conversion to Medicaid. Persons without economic resources were generally limited to less desirable places or to homes with long waiting lists.

Three years later, Peter's mother's condition deteriorated to the point that she required round-the-clock homecare by a nursing aide, which quickly depleted her reserves. This fact, and questions about the quality of care she was receiving, led Peter to apply to eight homes that he thought to be adequate facilities. Peter soon discovered, however, that because of a shortage of beds in the region, his mother's application was in competition with others who had greater economic assets. Three months later, as his mother's assets are approaching zero, he hopefully awaits word of acceptance. He has reached the point where he has become willing to guarantee one year of payment from his (formerly her) assets to increase his mother's chances of admission to a decent nursing home.

Case 3 — The Consequences of Innocence

Mary, a 50-year-old widow is, much to her surprise and dismay, homeless. For the past ten years, she and her teenage daughter shared a duplex with Mary's parents. Mary's income as a store clerk, coupled with her father's pension, had provided the family a relatively comfortable, but not extravagant life.

Three years ago, Mary's father suffered a stroke of sufficient severity that he required nursing-home care. His few savings were soon depleted and he went on Medicaid. Seven months later he died. Shortly thereafter Mary's mother became increasingly frail and confused. Eventually she too was placed in a nursing home under Medicaid. Last year, she died.

Sometime after the funeral, Mary was informed that the duplex, which she believed to be her own through inheritance, was to be confiscated by the state and sold at auction to defray the costs incurred by her parents' nursing home stays. Although Mary tried to get enough money together to buy the house, she was unsuccessful. To date she has had no luck finding an apartment of adequate size in a decent neighborhood that she can afford.

These three encounters with the Medicaid system suggest the diverse ways it influences the lives of the elderly and their families. Marilyn could not understand why Medicare, a health insurance program for the elderly, did not cover homecare and nursing-home care, services that are most likely to be needed by the aged. Nor could she understand the hospital's eagerness to discharge her mother without an acceptable discharge plan in that to her knowledge, Medicare did cover hospital care. She was overwhelmed by her limited choices of placing her mother in an apparently poor nursing home at the cost of her own economic independence, or of providing round-the-clock home care that was beyond her physical strength.

Peter, on the other hand, wonders how people without the economic assets to "buy in" to a decent nursing home manage to get their mothers into an acceptable facility. He also is concerned with the potential economic abuse children can impose on their parents as a result of a divestment. And, although Peter believes he had no choice but to circumvent the law, he does feel somewhat guilty knowing that he has violated the spirit, if not the letter, of Medicaid regulations. However, the relatively small amount of monies he controls as a result of divestment will be used according to his mother's wishes, to assist his own children financially.

Mary is bewildered and angry. She had no idea that spending down would result in the loss of what she always thought of as her home. She is particularly distressed because after her parents' retirement, she contributed substantial amounts of money to home maintenance and taxes in addition to paying off the remaining mortgage. Had she known, Mary would have had no qualms about changing legal ownership in order to protect the only major asset her parents ever had.

Cost Containment

The situations described above are in large measure the result of the recent radical shift in health care policy from expansion of entitlements and services to restrictions on service use. Since 1983, the federal government has been shifting a larger portion of health costs to Medicare beneficiaries and their families through greater use of services with co-insurance, use of services not covered by Medicare, and larger deductibles (for hospital care it was $400 per hospital stay in 1985 and $492 in 1986).

Homecare is also facing increasingly rigid eligibility guidelines. For example, although Medicare recipients must require "skilled" care, care only can be "intermittent" in kind, resulting in fewer visits per client.

Possibly the most radical cost-containment measure is the Medicare Prospective Payment System (PPS) that was implemented in 1983. PPS pays hospitals prospectively on the basis of a patient's classification in one of 468 Diagnostic-Related Groups (DRGs). The intent is for hospitals to increase revenues by decreasing patients' length of stay and use of hospital resources. But, as a result, older persons are being discharged earlier and with higher acuity levels than in the past, leading to an increased need for formal community homecare or for family care. The need for out-of-hospital care is of particular importance for women as they are less likely to have a spouse to provide informal homecare following hospital discharge. As a result, they must often rely on informal family care from children or turn to formal community homecare services that may not be affordable due to the limitations of Medicare coverage.

Prospective payment systems have also been implemented for Medicaid reimbursement of nursing-home care, as in the New York State Resource Utilization Group system. It is likely that other states will soon follow suit. One concern is that reimbursement categories adequately reflect service needs so that certain groups of elderly — for example, those with chronic mental disorders — are not discriminated against in admission policies because they bring in fewer dollars than others. Prospective payment systems for homecare are currently being tested and it is likely that they too will be implemented in the near future, decreasing access to homecare even further.

While cost-containment measures may be laudable attempts to assure that persons receive appropriate care from appropriate providers in a cost-effective manner, the difficulty is that such efforts reduce flexibility within the system. Thus if a particular service or type of care is not available or adequate at the time that it is needed, the system may not permit compensation for the use of other sources of care or assistance, even if only temporarily. Cost-containment measures do not recognize gaps in services such as inadequate Medicare coverage of nonprofessional homecare, day care, and respite services. Tightening access to existing services will underscore these deficiencies. As current cost-benefit formulas do not measure the health and social consequences of nonutilization of needed services, these consequences may not be evident in the statistics.

SUMMARY AND DISCUSSION

Poverty in old age is not simply an economic matter. It is too often associated with simultaneous "poverty" of health and "poverty" of freedom to make fundamental choices about the conditions under which one chooses to live during the last years of life. Women, especially women who are poor or who become poor as a result of age-related events such as widowhood and chronic illness, are at particular risk for such all-encompassing poverty. Currently, the social responses to this problem include Medicare, an insurance program, and Medicaid, a welfare program. While these programs are certainly better than having no insurance and welfare programs at all, gaps in Medicare coverage and the wide variation in Medicaid entitlements across states make old age a time of uncertainty for most Americans.

Current health-care policy for the elderly rests on the assumption that impoverishment is a precondition for receipt of publicly supported care, the same assumption that applies to those in younger age groups who receive public assistance. There is, however, a critical difference between the two groups. The young are poor because of their inability to engender income, for whatever reasons. They may qualify for a variety of social programs and strategies that hold potential for economic self-determination. The majority of elderly, on the other hand, are poor because of the age-related events of widowhood and illness, facts of life beyond the individual's and society's control. Older people inevitably face illness at some point in time between the onset of old age and death and the likelihood that the illness will be chronic and economically debilitating is greatest for women. The fact that women are most likely to experience illness-engendered poverty is a consequence of the privilege of long life, a privilege tempered by life-long economic inequality and old-age-related chronic illness.

The question that must be asked is whether chronic illness

should precipitate impoverishment for large numbers of older people as a result of their own illnesses or those of their spouses. Another issue is divestment. Divestment laws have been implemented in most states to prevent older persons from turning over their assets to others when it is clear that they need costly nursing-home care. Most laws require that assets must be diverted two or more years prior to Medicaid eligibility. These laws may serve only to delay the eventual divestment process and to bias evasion techniques in favor of those with access to legal information and counsel, that is, the well-off and those with the most to gain from "gaming" the system.

The difficult questions posed by illness-engendered poverty and by divestment arise in part from the absence of an equitable system of financing long-term care that would spread economic risk so that individuals are not impoverished as a result of old-age illness nor are motivated to "game" the system to prevent impoverishment. Welfare programs such as Medicaid that impoverish the working class while at the same time enable the wealthy to receive free life-long care from the state are fraught with problems.

The United States and the Republic of South Africa are the only two developed countries of the world that fail to provide a system of long-term care for their elderly citizens. One solution is a national health care system. Other "experiments" could include various types of long-term care insurance, reorientation of incentives from costly hospital and nursing-home care to comprehensive and articulated community-based services, and expansion of Medicare benefits. This is not to suggest that individuals not bear any responsibility for financing at least some of their own health care. For too many, however, health financing policies serve as an antecedent to poverty and poverty is far too often an antecedent to death.

REFERENCES

Berger, P. (1983). The economic well-being of elderly Hispanics. *Journal of Minority Aging,* 36-46.

Butler, R. N. & Newacheck, P. W. (1981). Health and social factors affecting long-term care policy. In J. Meltzer, F. Farrow & H. Richman *Policy Options in Long-term Care.* Chicago: University of Chicago Press.

Cantor, M. (1983). *Social care for the aged in the United States: Issues and challenges*. Reprint. New York: The Haworth Press, Inc.

Congressional Clearinghouse on the Future (1985). Tomorrow's elderly: *Issues for Congress*. Prepared for the House Select Committee on Aging: Congressional Institute for the Future.

Davis, K. (1986). What about the poor? *Generations, 9*, 13-15.

Davis, K., Gold, M. & Makuc, D. (1981). Access to health care for the poor: Does the gap remain? *Annual Review of Public Health, 2*, 159-182.

Harrington, C., Estes, C., Lee, P. & Newcomer, R. (1986). Effects of state Medicaid policies on the aged. *The Gerontologist, 26*, 437-443.

Holden, K. C., Burkhauser, R.V. & Myers, D.A. (1986). Income transitions at older stages of life: The dynamics of poverty. *The Gerontologist, 26*, 292-297.

Joe, T. C., Meltzer, J. & Yu, P. (1985). Arbitrary access to care: The case for reforming Medicaid. *Health Affairs, 4*, 59-74.

Kutza, E. (1981). *The benefits of old age*. Chicago: The University of Chicago Press.

Lehrman, R. (1980). Poverty statistics serve as nagging reminder. *Generations: Journal of the Western Gerontological Society, 4*, 17.

Nickman, J.R. (1986). Helping New York elders pay for long-term care: Opportunities for public-private cooperation. Prepared for *New York Affairs*. In press.

Palmore, E. B. (1986). Trends in the health of the aged. *The Gerontologist, 26*, 298-302.

Smeeding, T. M. (1986). Nonmoney income and the elderly: The case of the 'tweeners. *Journal of Policy Analysis and Management, 5*, 707-724.

Uhlenberg, P. & Salmon, M. P. (1986). Change in relative income of older women, 1960-1980. *The Gerontologist, 26*, 164-170.

U. S. Bureau of the Census (1985). Characteristics of the population below the poverty level: 1983. *Current Population Reports, Series P-60*, No. 147. Washington, DC: U.S. Government Printing Office.

U. S. Congress, Senate Special Committee on Aging (1983). *Developments in aging, 1983*. Washington, DC: Government Printing Office.

U. S. Congress, Senate Special Committee on Aging (1985). *Developments in aging, 1985*. Washington, DC: Government Printing Office.

U. S. Department of Health, Education, and Welfare (1983). *Income and resources of the aged*, Washington, DC: Government Printing Office.

U. S. Department of Health and Human Services (1984). *Long-term care financing and delivery systems: Exploring some alternatives*, (HCFA Publication No. 03174). Washington, DC: Government Printing Office.

U. S. Department of Health and Human Services (1985). *Monthly benefit statistics program data: Old-age survivors, disability, and health insurance*. Washington, DC: Government Printing Office.

Women's Equity Action League (WEAL) (1985). *Facts on Social Security*. Washington, DC: WEAL.

Changing Patterns of Health Insurance Coverage: Special Concerns for Women

James R. Tallon, Jr.
Rachel Block

SUMMARY. Health care expenditures and utilization have increased dramatically in recent years, but gaps in health insurance coverage restrict access to care for a growing portion of the population. Women are especially vulnerable given the structure of insurance coverage and demographic factors. The erosion of insurance coverage can be attributed to several trends, particularly employer cost containment strategies, restricted public program eligibility and changes in the characteristics of the work force. Numerous measures have been adopted at the federal and state levels to maintain or expand coverage on an incremental basis. As broader segments of the population suffer reduction or loss of coverage, a comprehensive approach will be necessary to ensure universal access to health care.

Health care expenditures and utilization have undergone tremendous growth in recent years; in 1984, total expenditures reached almost $400 billion, or 11 percent of the gross national product (Levit et al., 1985). Factors that have contributed to this growth include dramatic increases in the supply of health care providers, widespread availability of private health insurance, establishment of major publicly financed and administered programs including Medicare and Medicaid, and the rapid development of new medical technologies. These increased costs have

---

James R. Tallon, Jr., is Majority Leader, New York State Assembly and previously served as Chairman, Committee on Health. Rachel Block is Study Director, Subcommittee on Health Insurance, New York State Council on Health Care Financing.

119

become a major concern of private and public payers and have led to the development of a wide variety of measures to control costs and utilization.

For a significant and growing portion of the population, however, the benefits of the health care boom have not been realized due to gaps in health insurance coverage. The uninsured and underinsured are a diverse and changing group whose characteristics cut across income levels, age, gender and employment status. Women are particularly vulnerable given the structure of insurance coverage in relation to employment, demographic factors, and their particular health care needs.

Gaining access to health care services has become increasingly difficult for those who do not have adequate coverage, and a number of trends will result in further restrictions in the immediate future. Policy responses to deal with these critical concerns must take into account the dimensions of the problem and trends affecting the availability and cost of coverage. Discrete measures aimed at the populations in need must be merged to form a complete system of health insurance coverage.

DIMENSIONS OF THE PROBLEM

Precise measures of the uninsured and underinsured are not available, but there is sufficient data to generally describe the nature and scope of the problem. In 1984 approximately 35 million people, 17 percent of the total population, lacked health insurance (Sulvetta & Swartz, 1986). In 1977, a comprehensive survey estimated that 27 million, 13 percent of the population, were uninsured (Kaspar et al., undated). In addition, depending on the definition used, approximately the same number of people are underinsured (i.e., risk significant financial burden due to gaps in coverage or cost-sharing requirements under existing insurance) (Farley, 1985a).

Patterns of coverage vary widely based on factors including income, sex, age, type of employment/employment status and geographic location. Slightly more than one-half of the uninsured population had family income below 150 percent of the poverty level in 1984; 12.6 million (35.6 percent) were below poverty;

and 5.9 million (16.7 percent) had incomes of 100-149 percent of poverty. Children made up one-third of the uninsured. Two-thirds of uninsured children lived in poor and near-poor families; more than half lived in two-parent households, while 38 percent lived in female-headed households. This pattern differs from the overall distribution of poor children, one half of whom live in female-headed households (U.S. Bureau of Census, 1985). Yet women were as likely to be covered as men according to the 1977 survey, and the 1984 data indicate roughly the same number in each group are uninsured (11.9 million men compared to 11.4 million women) (Sulvetta & Swartz, 1986).

Private Coverage

Private sources of insurance covered about 65 percent of the total population (Walden et al., 1985). Most private coverage is provided through employment-related groups. Individual-purchase insurance represents only a small but important percentage. However, employment-based coverage is not uniformly available. Based on 1984 data, over half of the uninsured, 56.5 percent, were employed on a full- or part-time basis, and 12 percent were unemployed (i.e., not working but still in the labor force) (Sulvetta and Swartz, 1986).

In 1980, full-time workers accounted for almost 40 percent of the uninsured, while part-time workers represented 17 percent of the total. The dependents of employed persons were an important component as well: children made up 20 percent of this group, while spouses added another 10 percent. In total, over three-quarters of the uninsured population is made up of employed persons and their dependents (Monheit et al., 1985).

The employed uninsured are heterogeneous. One-third are young (ages 19-24) but older, full-time workers account for approximately one-half of the total. Small firms are much less likely to offer coverage, extend coverage to dependents or contribute a significant portion of the insurance premium. In addition, employment-based coverage is less prevalent in the agriculture, construction and services industries, as compared to professional and manufacturing jobs (Monheit et al., 1985).

Variations in employment-based coverage are particularly apparent among women. Women are more likely to work in small firms, services industries and temporary jobs where insurance coverage and other benefits are less likely to be offered. Slightly more than half of female household heads had private coverage, compared to over 80 percent of male household heads. This pattern is consistent for full-time and part-time workers, as well as for persons who are not employed — differences range from 10-25 percent when comparing male and female household heads (Farley, 1985b). Age-related differences are also significant. Based on a special tabulation of 1984 data of women aged 15-44, almost 30 percent of women aged 18-24 had no coverage, while 65 percent had private coverage. Of women aged 30-44, only 11 percent were uninsured, while 85 percent had private insurance (Gold & Kenney, 1985).

Public Coverage

Medicare and Medicaid are the major publicly administered and financed programs, providing comprehensive health insurance coverage to the elderly and the poor, respectively. Each program has made significant strides in expanding coverage within these populations, but coverage is by no means complete in terms of target populations and services covered.

Medicare covers almost all persons aged 65 and over and accounts for 12 percent of the total population's coverage (Walden et al., 1985). However, due to cost-sharing requirements and service restrictions and exclusions, Medicare actually covers less than half of the elderly's total health care costs (see Grau, this volume; Davis & Rowland, 1986). Long-term, custodial care and outpatient prescription drugs are important services for many elderly persons, but neither is eligible for Medicare reimbursement. Because of the elderly's income profile, out-of-pocket health care expenses can be a barrier to needed care and a significant financial burden; a growing number of the elderly are forced into poverty due to health care expenses.

Women currently account for 60 percent of Medicare enrollees (Gornick et al., 1985), proportional to their representation in the 65 and older population, but there are major differences between men and women within this group. Women are much more likely to be widowed or single (60 percent of those aged 65 and older, 76 percent of those aged 75 and older) (Davis & Rowland, 1986). Elderly women are also more likely to be poor since women account for three-quarters of the elderly poor population (Minkler & Stone, 1985). There are numerous causes, but gaps in Medicare coverage are partially responsible for the higher rate of impoverishment: women generally live longer, suffer from more chronic conditions, and often lack the support systems necessary to live independently, leading to greater need for institutional services that rapidly deplete one's financial resources.

According to Walden et al., (1985). Medicaid accounts for 10 percent of total coverage available, but there are major gaps in coverage of the poor population it was intended to serve. Some groups are "categorically" eligible, while others may be covered at the discretion of individual states. Some services are mandated for coverage, while others are optional; one state offers four optional services, while another offers 29 (Desonia & King, 1985). Income eligibility criteria also vary widely among states. As a result it is estimated that less than 50 percent of the total poor population is covered by Medicaid. In individual states, as little as 23 percent or as much of 97 percent of the poor population may be covered (U.S. Department of Health and Human Services, 1983).

Medicaid eligibility restrictions have a significant impact on poor women, particularly female heads of households. Among women aged 15-44 with incomes below the poverty level, 40 percent received Medicaid and 36 percent had no insurance coverage; for incomes at 100-149 percent of the poverty level, 10 percent were receiving Medicaid and 30 percent had no insurance coverage (Gold & Kenney, 1985). In addition, Medicaid is an important safety net for elderly poor women, but a significant number are denied coverage for their non-Medicare health expenses due to income and other eligibility restrictions.

To summarize, the combination of private and public insurance coverage provides an extensive base of protection, but a significant number of people are uninsured or underinsured. The population is diverse, but women – particularly the poor and near-poor – are disproportionately represented among the uninsured. The dimensions of the problem are especially alarming in view of the consequences: restricted access to health care services and ensuing deteriorating health status.

INSURANCE COVERAGE, HEALTH STATUS AND UTILIZATION

The significance of gaps in health insurance coverage can be measured in terms of its implications for health status, utilization and financial burdens placed on individuals and health care providers. The impact goes beyond the unnecessary personal hardship placed on individuals since society ultimately shares the cost of reduced economic productivity, uncompensated care and greater severity or complexity of illness resulting from deferred care. With health insurance the primary means of financing one's health care expenses, gaps in coverage are likely to restrict access to care, particularly among the poor and low-income population. These gaps will also strain the financial stability of health care providers serving the medically indigent. Both of these phenomena have been amply documented.

Health Status and Utilization

The uninsured are more likely to report poorer health status, but it is not clear how these variables interact. Health status may cause lack of coverage due to employment barriers or the eligibility and underwriting practices of insurance companies. On the other hand, lack of insurance may contribute to poorer health status because of deferred or denied care. Both variables correlate with the general socioeconomic profile of the uninsured.

The uninsured also report less utilization of physician and hospital services. One major study found that insured persons used 50 percent more ambulatory care and 90 percent more hospital services than the uninsured. For those reporting poorer health status, the insured reported 70 percent more ambulatory care utilization (Davis & Roland, 1983). A recent national survey of persons without insurance found that they were three times more likely not to get health care services when needed (Robert Wood Johnson Foundation, 1983).

More detailed, epidemiological evidence is available from recent studies conducted in California and Arizona. Medically indigent adults terminated from California's Medicaid program were studied at six-month and one-year intervals following termination. Sixty-nine percent of the group were women, with average monthly income ranging from $250-500 (annual $3000-6000), and most suffered from one or more chronic conditions, such as hypertension and diabetes. Access to care and health status had diminished significantly during the study period despite transfer of responsibility for medically indigent care to the counties (Lurie et al., 1984; Lurie et al., 1986).

The Arizona study compared access among low-income people in that state before the establishment of its Medicaid program with the rest of the country. There was significantly reduced physician utilization among the Arizona residents, particularly children. In addition, low-income persons in Arizona were twice as likely to report that care had been refused to a family member due to lack of coverage or inability to pay. During this time, Arizona's medically indigent were also served by public clinics and other providers as uncompensated care costs (Blendon et al., 1986). These studies may demonstrate the importance of insurance coverage in obtaining care as compared to provider-based approaches.

One area in which access barriers for low-income women are particularly apparent is prenatal, maternal and infant care. Adequate prenatal care is an important determinant of health for both mother and infant. In 1982, 5 percent of all pregnant women received very late (third trimester) or no prenatal care while 18 percent did not receive prenatal care until the second trimester (Gold & Kenney, 1985). Lack of insurance coverage clearly plays a role in delayed prenatal services, which has been directly linked to complications in pregnancy and low birth weight, each of which pose significant health risks.

Even women with coverage may face barriers to care since insurance policies may not provide comprehensive coverage for maternal/infant care, and Medicaid fee schedules are substantially below standard charges, which limits physicians' willingness to serve pregnant Medicaid recipients. However, lack of any health insurance coverage is far more likely to impede access to adequate prenatal and infant services than is inadequate insurance.

Uncompensated care plays an important role in the provision of health services to the uninsured and underinsured population. These costs have a significant financial impact on providers, particularly hospitals. Total uncompensated care (representing both bad debts and charity care) was estimated at $6.2 billion in 1982, or 6 percent of total hospital revenues. The burden of providing such care is disproportionately borne by certain types of facilities, generally teaching hospitals and public hospitals (Sloan et al., 1986).

According to Sloan et al.' study (1986), pregnancy-related care, mostly deliveries, accounts for a substantial portion of uncompensated care costs. Deliveries made up 40 percent of the discharges and one-quarter of the estimated costs in the self-pay/no-charge category (almost synonymous with "uncompensated care"). This is not the only index by which to assess low-income women's access to services, but given the severe data limitations, maternal/infant care can be viewed as an indicator of broader access problems resulting from lack of insurance coverage.

TRENDS IN AVAILABILITY AND COST OF COVERAGE

Patterns of health insurance coverage evolve from a complex web of interacting trends in both the private and public domains. While there are many direct and indirect factors affecting the availability and costs of coverage, the most fundamental relate to shifts in employment patterns, employers' cost-containment strategies, changes in reimbursement policies, and trends in Medicaid eligibility and utilization. Several of these basic elements have direct consequences for uninsured poor and low-income women.

Employment Patterns

Two major trends in employment patterns will have a significant impact on employment-based health insurance coverage, particularly in relation to women. First, the shift from manufacturing and other goods-producing industries to services industries (retail trade, business services, health care, communications) will affect the overall distribution of employment-based coverage. Many of the high-growth categories of industries and occupations also have the lowest percentage of group health or pension coverage. Among services occupations, approximately one-third of employees have group health insurance, compared to almost 80 percent of professional and managerial employees and two-thirds to three-quarters of workers in goods-producing occupations. Retail trade, business services and personal services cover 38 percent, 49 percent and 22 percent of employees, respectively, compared to manufacturing (82 percent) transportation/utilities (81 percent) and professional (61 percent) categories (U.S. Bureau of the Census, 1984).

Second, there has been tremendous growth in the temporary/part-time employment sectors. This shift is related to the growth in services industries, but it also reflects broader phenomena such as increasing numbers of women in the work force and employers' efforts to reduce fringe-benefit commitments. It is estimated that up to 30 million people, about one-quarter of the work force, are represented in this growing employment category (see Stellman, this volume). Since part-time workers already constitute a significant portion of the uninsured population, this shift in economic structure will expand the number of persons without health insurance coverage.

Employer Cost-Containment Initiatives

In a 1984 survey of over 1,000 firms offering group benefits, 97 percent indicated that they had changed their health plans in response to increased health care expenditures and almost two-thirds had implemented five or more cost-containment provisions. The most common approach has been to change employee behavior with respect to utilization, accomplished largely through measures shifting costs to employees (e.g., increased deductibles, copayments and employee contributions for self- and dependent coverage) (Employee Benefit Research Institute, 1986).

While cost-sharing is intended to reduce utilization of services and increase consumers' cost-consciousness in relation to health care, it also may result in delaying necessary care, thereby increasing long-term expenditures. Research findings on this issue are inconclusive, but it is clear that increasing employees' costs will have a disproportionate impact on persons with low income and/or poor health status. In addition, increased employee costs for dependent coverage would further reduce the base of coverage among spouses and children of employed persons, already a significant component of the uninsured population.

A more radical form of cost control may be to curtail or terminate retiree health benefits. The U.S. Department of Labor has estimated employers' unfunded liability for retiree health benefits at $98 billion according to a *New York Times* report (Greenhouse, 1986). A business-group survey indicated that only 5 percent of respondent companies pre-fund their retiree health plans (Cronin & Amkraut, 1985). In cases of bankruptcy and corporate restructuring, both increasingly prevalent, retirees are at substantial risk for loss or drastic reduction of their health insurance coverage. Congress recently considered mandating employer pre-funding for insurance, but the costs associated with such a mandate may result in further benefits restrictions for this already-vulnerable population. Reduced employer commitments to retiree benefits will inevitably increase reliance on Medicare, Medicaid and other mechanisms, thereby placing greater demands on the already-strained resources. This shift would necessitate commitment of additional public resources or redistribution of existing program funds.

Changes in Hospital Reimbursement Policies

Part of the private and public sector cost-containment strategy has been to modify hospital-reimbursement practices. Until recently, hospitals had considerable latitude in determining charges for various services according to payer. This discretion was widely used to cross-subsidize services for which there was inadequate or no payment. Thus, some portion of a hospital's uncompensated care burden would be financed through higher charges (Phelps, 1986). Government and private payers have moved away from retrospective payment of charges to prospective payment based on costs, capitation formulae or negotiated rates. As a result, the costs associated with uncompensated care have become isolated and payers are no longer willing to share them.

Services provided by hospitals to the uninsured and underinsured are an important component of access to health care for this impoverished population. Historical reimbursement practices may not have been equitable, but the hidden subsidy represented by an unspoken consensus on addressing the problem through cross-subsidies provided a financing mechanism. Erosion of this mechanism comes at a time when the uninsured population is growing and hospitals are operating in a more competitive environment, reducing their ability to fund uncompensated care through such indirect means. Several states have recently enacted programs to finance uncompensated hospital-care costs explicitly through a variety of financing mechanisms such as taxes on hospital revenues or on insurance premiums (Desonia & King, 1985). However, these measures are limited in scope and availability.

Trends in Medicaid Eligibility and Utilization

There are many forces operating simultaneously at the federal and state levels both to constrict and to expand the Medicaid program. In general, the early 1980s were characterized by eligibility and service restrictions. More recent legislative efforts have focused on restoring those cuts and expanding program commitments in limited ways. At the same time, Medicaid program expenditures have shifted to more long-term care, with little growth and a proportionate decline in primary care expenditures. Since Medicaid is a critical source of coverage for poor women, these trends are particularly relevant to their insurance status.

Eligibility

In 1981, the federal Omnibus Budget Reconciliation Act (OBRA) reduced matching payments to states and restricted AFDC eligibility criteria, particularly for working-poor women. Almost one-half million cases were terminated, resulting for most in termination of Medicaid eligibility. A net loss of 600,000 Medicaid recipients between 1981 and 1983 can be directly attributed to the OBRA cuts (Mundinger, 1985). U.S. General Accounting Office (1985) found that in selected site studies "the typical working recipient who lost benefits—indeed the typical AFDC case—was a women about 30 years old with two children"; one-half had no private coverage available after termination from Medicaid.

There has also been considerable activity at the state level. During 1981, more than 30 states enacted reductions or limitations in their Medicaid programs. At the same time, a small number expanded eligibility for targeted groups. A shift to structural reforms began in 1982, when only three states reduced eligibility and 14 adopted eligibility-expansion measures. By 1984, federal legislation was adopted which required states to cover children and pregnant women under certain circumstances, and states responded by expanding eligibility for these and other groups. From 1983 through 1985, a total of 70 state laws were enacted to expand eligibility (Intergovernmental Health Policy Project 1982, 1983, 1985). However, these measures may have served only to reinstate persons terminated during 1981-82 and to have kept up with growth in the poverty population. Recent data suggest that total Medicaid enrollment increased by 600,000 from 1982 through 1984, a figure similar to the net reduction reported earlier.

Utilization

Medicaid has increasingly become a long-term care financing program for Supplemental Security Income (SSI) recipients and elderly persons impoverished by chronic-care costs. In 1984, of those categorically eligible for Medicaid, two-thirds were eligible through AFDC (by definition, mostly poor women and children), accounting for one-quarter of total expenditures. SSI recipients made up one-quarter of the recipient population but consumed 72 percent of the service costs (Levit et al., 1985). These figures underestimate Medicaid's coverage of the elderly since 25 percent qualify through medically needy programs (compared to 11 percent of the under 65 population). The medically needy aged account for 45 percent of the total Medicaid expenditures for elderly persons; one-quarter of the medically needy aged used skilled nursing facilities, compared to 5 percent of Medicaid's cash assistance elderly (Davis & Rowland, 1986).

These phenomena pose a serious dilemma to coverage of poor and low-income women since increased costs associated with elderly women severely constrain resources available to serve younger women and children. Projected demographic trends indicate a significant increase in the elderly population. In the absence of alternative long-term care financing measures for this group, the resource-consumption patterns will intensify fiscal pressures on Medicaid serving all the various components of the poor and near-poor population.

CLOSING THE GAPS

It is apparent that major gaps in health insurance coverage affect millions of Americans, impede access to necessary health care and seriously affect health and well-being. Current patterns of coverage have resulted from a wide variety of forces. The public sector has assumed a major role in expanding coverage for high-risk populations — the elderly and the poor — but its commitment expands or contracts over time, and universal health insurance coverage remains an elusive policy objective.

Financing uncompensated care and expanding the availability of insurance have recently emerged as priority concerns at the federal and state levels. As a result, various measures that respond to specific components of the problem have been adopted. These approaches generally fall into three categories: insurance approaches, provider subsidies, and Medicaid and indigent-care program expansion. Poor and low-income women can benefit from all of these initiatives.

Insurance Approaches

Federal and state laws have recently been enacted which require continuation of employees' group health insurance for specified periods of time if employment is terminated. Provisions of the federal Consolidated Omnibus Budget Reconciliation Act of 1985 (COBRA) require continued coverage at a premium not to exceed 102 percent of the group rate. Continuation must be offered for 18 months in cases of employment termination and 36 months in cases of the employee's death, divorce or separation, eligibility for Medicare, or loss of dependent child status. As of 1985, more than 20 states had enacted continued coverage statutes applying to employment termination and/or layoff (Desonia & King, 1985; King, personal communication). Group premiums are much less expensive than individual-purchase insurance, and waiting periods or restrictions on preexisting conditions are prohibited under a continued policy. Thus, such mandated continuation laws represent a significant protection for employees and insured dependents.

Certain types and levels of benefits are frequently required under state laws as well. Mandated benefits assure a minimum level of coverage, thus partially addressing access problems for particular services. Coverage for care of newborns is required in all states, and maternity coverage is mandated in 38 states (Clearinghouse on Business Coalitions, 1985). The federal Pregnancy Discrimination Act of 1978 also requires employers to cover maternity care in the same manner as other health services. However, levels of coverage vary considerably, so the insured person's financial exposure may still be significant (Gold & Kenney, 1985).

Insurance mandates can be effective under a narrow range of circumstances, but there is little interstate uniformity and increased costs may deter employers from providing any health insurance coverage at all. Federal law prohibits states from regulating self-insured health plans, so many employers have taken the route of self-insurance to avoid state-mandated insurance requirements. State mandates regarding certain conditions of coverage may in some cases be counterproductive in the absence of federal requirements.

Provider Subsidies

Direct payments to providers do not expand the base of insurance coverage but they are an important means of improving access to health services for the medically indigent. Among the major initiatives in this category are state programs that reimburse providers, primarily hospitals, for some portion of uncompensated care costs. Several states include subsidies directly in hospital reimbursement rates, while others pool funds derived from reimbursement rate "add-ons" or hospital revenue assessments. A few states mandate a prescribed level of "charity" care as a condition for the institution to operate and do not provide additional resources (Desonia & King, 1985).

There are numerous shortcomings associated with provider subsidy programs. Ensuring access to institutional services does not provide comprehensive primary care for the uninsured. It is also difficult to monitor and enforce a particular level of "charity care" in return for additional payment, leading to reduced accountability for these expenditures. The distribution of costs associated with financing uncompensated care programs may be arbitrary or inequitable, and hospitals or insurers may resist statutory "add-ons" or assessments. While this approach can help assure a minimum level of institutional services, it is a narrow and uncertain financing mechanism and does not expand the base of coverage.

Medicaid and Indigent Care Program Expansion

A simple and direct means of expanding coverage for the poor would be to standardize Medicaid eligibility criteria among the states and to set income eligibility at the federal poverty level. In the present budgetary climate, such a proposal may not be realistic. Congress, however, enacted legislation this year authorizing states to increase Medicaid eligibility for pregnant women and infants, and elderly persons, with incomes up to the poverty level (U.S. Congress, 1986).

Several states have enacted major indigent-care programs targeted to particular groups or services. Texas, South Carolina, New York and Florida are among the states that have recently initiated or expanded major indigent care programs, particularly targeted to prenatal and infant care services. Several states have developed programs to assist low income elderly persons in financing prescription drug costs (Bazzoli, 1985). While Medicaid eligibility provides a comprehensive range of services, these new programs try to use limited state resources to serve priority needs for portions of the non-Medicaid, low-income population. State indigent care programs serve important needs, but they will not be able to cover all of the medically indigent.

PROSPECTS FOR THE FUTURE

Given the scope and diverse nature of the problem, the measures described above will not be sufficient to provide comprehensive coverage for the uninsured and underinsured. Major structural changes would be necessary to remedy the problem, which is continuing to expand under present arrangements. A broad-based national health insurance program could build on the current base of coverage through mandated employee and dependents benefits and full coverage of poor persons under Medicaid. A long-term care component could be added to the present Medicare program, thereby alleviating a significant (and unwarranted) burden on Medicaid dollars.

The informal and incomplete responses that currently exist can no longer be relied on for the millions of people who are disenfranchised from the emerging health-care system. Poor and low income women are particularly at risk for declining health and for further financial devastation if gaps in health insurance coverage are not closed in a timely and comprehensive manner. The public and private sectors must share responsibility for financing a system that assures access to health care according to need, not income, gender or age. The cost will be substantial, but failure to act will result in significant human and fiscal consequences.

The persistent erosion of health insurance coverage is a growing problem. While many of those affected are poor and low-income, gaps in coverage now extend to all segments of the population. The breadth and complexity of factors contributing to trends in coverage will require more sweeping actions, and involve a broader range of constituencies, than past efforts directed to the poor. Thus a unique opportunity exists to mobilize divergent groups on behalf of the measures needed to establish health insurance coverage for the entire population.

REFERENCES

Bazzoli, G. (1985). *Health care for the indigent: Literature review and research agenda for the future*. Chicago: American Hospital Association.

Blendon, R., Aiken, L., Freeman, H., Kirkman-Liff, B. & Murphy, J. (1986). Uncompensated care by hospitals or public insurance for the poor, Does it make a difference? *New England Journal of Medicine, 314*, 1160-63.

Clearinghouse on Business Coalition for Health Action (1985). *Coalition Report, 4* (7), 3.

Cronin, C. & Amkraut, C. (1985). *Retiree health benefits: Issues and options*. Washington, DC: Washington Business Group on Health.

Davis, K. and Rowland, D. (1983). Uninsured and underserved: Inequities in health care in the United States. *Milbank Memorial Fund Quarterly, 61* (2), 160-66.

Davis, K. & Rowland, D. (1986). *Medicare policy: New directions for health and long-term care*. Baltimore: John Hopkins University.

Desonia, R. & King, K. (1985). *State programs of assistance for the medically indigent*. Washington, DC: Intergovernmental Health Policy Project.

Employee Benefit Research Institute (1986). Private initiatives to contain health care expenditures. *EBRI Issue Brief*, (55), 5-6.

Farley, P. (1985a). Who are the uninsured? *Milbank Memorial Fund Quarterly, 63* (3). 477.

Farley, P. (1985b). *Private insurance and public programs: Coverage of health services, data preview 20*. Rockville, MD: U.S. Department of Health and Human Services.

Gold, R.B. & Kinney, A. (1985). Paying for maternity care. *Family Planning Perspectives, 17* (3), 105.

Gornick, M., Greenberg, J., Eggers, P. & Dobson, A. (1985). Twenty years of Medicare and Medicaid: Covered population, use of benefits and program expenditures. *Health Care Financing Review*, Annual Supplement.

Greenhouse, S. (1986). Health plans are feeling a little peaked. *New York Times*, August 24, 1986, E5.

Intergovernmental Health Policy Project (1982, 1983). *Recent and proposed changes in state Medicaid programs: A fifty state survey*. Washington, DC: Intergovernmental Health Policy Project.

Intergovernmental Health Policy Project (1985). *Major changes in state Medicaid and indigent care programs*. Washington, DC: Intergovernmental Health Policy Project.

Kaspar, J., Walden, D. & Wilensky, G. (undated). *Who are the uninsured? Data preview 1*. Hyattsville, MD: U.S. Department of Health and Human Services.

Levit, K., Lazenby, H., Waldo, D. & Davidoff, L. (1985). National health expenditures, 1984. *Health Care Financing Review, 7* (1), 1.

Lurie, N., Ward, N., Shapiro, M. & Brook, R. (1984). Termination from Medi-Cal — Does it affect health? *New England Journal of Medicine, 311* (7), 480-84.

Lurie, N., Ward, N., Shapiro, M., Gallego, C., Vaghaiwalla, R. & Brook, R. (1986). Termination of Medi-Cal benefits, A follow-up study one year later. *New England Journal of Medicine, 314* (19), 1266-68.

Minkler, M. & Stone, R. (1985). The feminization of poverty and older women. *The Gerontologist, 25* (4), 352.

Monheit, A., Hagan, M., Berk, M. & Farley, P. (1985). The employed uninsured and the role of public policy. *Inquiry, 22,* 349.

Mundinger, M. 0. (1985). Health service funding cuts and the declining health of the poor. *New England Journal of Medicine, 313* (1), 45.

Phelps, C. (1986). Cross-subsidies and charge-shifting in American hospitals. In Sloan, F., Blumstein, J. & Perrin, J. (Eds.) *Uncompensated hospital care: Rights and responsibilities* (pp. 19-24). Baltimore: John Hopkins University Press.

Robert Wood Johnson Foundation (1983). *Updated report on access to health care for the American people.* Princeton: Robert Wood Johnson Foundation.

Sloan, F., Valvona, J. & Mullner, R. (1986). Identifying the issues: A statistical profile. In F. Sloan, J. Blumstein and J. Perrin (Eds.) *Uncompensated hospital care: Rights and responsibilities* (pp. 19-24). Baltimore: John Hopkins University Press.

Sulvetta, M. & Swartz, K. (1986). *The uninsured and uncompensated care: A chartbook.* Washington, DC: National Health Policy Forum.

U.S. Bureau of the Census (1985). Characteristics of the population below the poverty level: 1983. *Current Population Reports,* Series P. 60, No. 147.

U.S. Bureau of the Census (1984). Employees with employer- or union-provided pension plans or groups health plans, by occupation and industry: 1982. *Statistical Abstract of the United States 1985.* Washington, DC: U.S. Government Printing Office.

U.S. Congress (1986). PL 99-509 (HR5300).

U.S. Department of Health and Human Services (1983). *The Medicare and Medicaid data book,* 1983. Baltimore: U.S. Department of Health and Human Services.

U.S. General Accounting Office (1985). *An evaluation of the 1981 AFDC changes: Final report.* Washington, DC: U.S. General Accounting Office.

Walden, D., Wilensky, G. & Kaspar, J. (1985). *Changes in health insurance status: Full year and part year coverage, data preview 21.* Rockville, MD: U.S. Department of Health and Human Services.

A Research Agenda on Issues Affecting Poor and Minority Women: A Model for Understanding Their Health Needs

Ruth E. Zambrana, PhD

SUMMARY. Acquiring data on quality of life indicators such as health, mental health and family roles of poor and minority women remains a low research priority. This paper provides an assessment of current knowledge in this area and an overview of the context in which poor and racial/ethnic women utilize health care services. A model that encompasses the interactive effects of race, gender and class variables is proposed. Such a model is a necessity for understanding the health needs of poor and racial/ethnic women. Suggestions for future research and policy formulation are given.

INTRODUCTION

The major purposes of this paper are threefold: to provide an assessment of current knowledge on the health of poor and racial/ethnic women; to present an overview of the context of their use of health services; and to propose a research agenda and a model for understanding their health needs. While the particular needs of women in general have generated serious concern and stimulated research on women's issues in the last decade, the needs of the most disadvantaged sectors of the population, poor women

Ruth E. Zambrana is affiliated with the School of Social Welfare, University of California, 247E Dodd Hall, Los Angeles, CA 90024.

The author acknowledges the support of a UCLA Faculty Career Development award during the Fall, 1986 for preparation of this manuscript. Further acknowledgment is made to the research and editorial assistance of Laura Cummins and Robert Wymss.

and women of color[1] have not received as extensive attention. The quality of life of poor and minority women, with specific reference to their health, mental health and family roles, has been a low research priority. Rather, the majority of studies have focused either on the cultural consequences of their behavior or on issues related to acculturation into the dominant society (see reviews by Andrade, 1983; Baca-Zinn, 1982). Most studies also have tended to ignore issues of class (Nelson, 1982). Only a limited number of studies, mainly qualitative or of small sample size, and essays have attempted to identify special health needs of Latina and Black women (Boone, 1982; Jackson, 1981; Melville, 1980; Zambrana (ed.), 1982).

Although research has suggested that poor and racial/ethnic women face many social and economic barriers in their attempts to integrate into the dominant culture and that their health status is poor, the interpretations of the findings have led to explanations such as culture as an explanatory variable that have not significantly contributed to our knowledge of this group. Traditional, rigid demarcations between investigations of health and mental status and those of work and family roles have generated a limited model of women's health. More recently, researchers have developed a keener awareness of the relationship between work and family roles and health and mental health status (Kanter, 1977; Nathanson, 1980; Zambrana & Hurst, 1984). For poor and racial/ethnic women in particular, these relationships have become strikingly clear as women's role responsibilities have increased. The socioeconomic dimensions, including multiple role responsibilities within the family and psychosocial factors such as chronic life stress and forms of social support, are critical to an understanding of the health status of poor and minority women.

BACKGROUND CHARACTERISTICS OF POOR AND MINORITY WOMEN

A review of the socio-demographic characteristics of the poor[2] and racial/ethnic[3] populations helps to explain some of the socioeconomic realities that influence their health status and other quality-of-life indicators. Blacks and Hispanics in the United States constitute about 18% of the total U.S. population. Blacks, the largest racial/ethnic minority group in the U.S., are predominately concentrated in the South (53%) and in large urban centers in the Northeast and Northcentral regions of the U.S. Seventynine percent of Blacks have completed high school and 13% are college graduates. The median income of Black families in 1981 was $13,270. Blacks are highly concentrated in service occupations (23%); as operators and laborers (27%); and as administrative support staff (24%). The Black unemployment rate is currently 18.9% (USDHHS, 1985a).

The 14.6 million Hispanics in the United States represent 6.4% of the total U.S. population.[4] The largest group is comprised of Mexican-Americans (60%), concentrated in the Southwest, followed by Puerto Ricans (14%) in the Northeast. In the past 15 years there has been a large influx of immigrants from Cuba (6%), South America and, most recently, Central America (20%). Geographically, 86% of all Hispanics live within ten states and 63% are concentrated in three states: California, Texas and New York. The great majority live in urban areas (U.S. Subcommittee on Census and Population, 1983).

Income potential is greatly affected by education. Lack of education clearly diminishes opportunities in the labor market. Hispanics tend to have completed fewer median school years than the general population. They also tend to be concentrated in lower-status blue-collar and white-collar occupations. Fifty-eight percent of Hispanics have completed a high school education. The median number of school years completed for Mexican-American women is 8.8 years; for Puerto Rican women it is 9.9 years; and for other Hispanics it is 12.2 years. For Black women, the median number of school years completed is 12.1 years. Education trends today for Black and Latina women continue to lag far behind white women (Johnson, 1984; Massey, 1982).

Black, Mexican-American and Puerto Rican women also tend to have more children at earlier ages than Anglo women and women in other Hispanic groups. The fertility rates for Puerto Rican, Mexican-American and Black women are the same, 2.3 births per woman, compared to a rate of 1.7 for nonminority women. Just over half (51%) of Spanish-origin women and nearly half of Black women (49.4%) have incomes below the poverty level, compared with one-fourth (25.7%) of Anglo women. The poverty rate for Latino heads of household is 3.4 times greater than that for whites. For Puerto Rican, 40% of families are headed by women, compared to 37.7% of Blacks. For Mexican-Americans and other Hispanic families, the female head-of-household rates are about one-half these figures: 16% and 18%, respectively. The real income of Hispanic female-headed families declined during the 1970s (U.S. Commission on Civil Rights, 1982).

Women, especially racial/ethnic women, are also at a disadvantage because of the inability to find work and lower earnings. If wives and female heads of household were paid the wages that similarly qualified men received, about half of the families now living in poverty would no longer be poor. Currently, the incomes of more than one-third of single mothers with children under six who work full-time at paid labor are still below the poverty line (Pearce & McAdoo, 1981:3).

FACTORS THAT CONTRIBUTE TO HEALTH STATUS: CURRENT KNOWLEDGE

A major effort to address substantive and research issues in the area of women's health was realized at a conference sponsored by the National Center for Health Services Research. One major theme of the presented papers was:

> . . . the worlds of women as relatives of the ill, as patients themselves or as decision-makers in situations influencing the health and health care of workers should be analyzed with respect to and for the meanings held by women in those worlds. In sum, research about women must be grounded in women's views, definitions, and concerns lest health care research continue to render inaccurate and biased views of those worlds based on the inappropriate categories generated at second hand by persons not a part of those worlds. (Olesen, 1977, p. 2)

Unfortunately, conference participants limited themselves to addressing a homogeneous population. As one commentator aptly pointed out, "we spent relatively little time delineating in specific terms the kinds of research needed to identify the needs of different segments of the female population—the racial segments, the ethnic segments, the children, the older women" (Olesen, 1977).

A later analysis of "areas of deficient data collection and integration," related to womens health failed to even mention the need to collect data on minority women or other subpopulations (Mueller, 1979). Information on the health status of poor and minority women, particularly their utilization patterns and help-seeking behaviors, are sorely lacking. A review of data in *Women and Health, U.S. 1980* (Moore, 1980) advised, in one paragraph, that data on minority women are needed.

Since the late 1970s there have been a number of data-collection efforts that have provided national data on racial/ethnic minorities. The undercount of the Black and Hispanic populations in the 1970 Census led to political advocacy by representatives of these groups to obtain national data. The 1978 National Health Interview Survey was the first effort to obtain data on a representative sample of the Black population. The National Health Interview Survey (Trevino & Moss, 1984) and the Hispanic Health and Nutrition Examination Survey (HHANES) represent national data-collection efforts resulting from several years of political advocacy on the part of Hispanic organizations.

During the last decade there have been three major government reports on the health status of low-income and minority populations. Health status trends among these groups were first substantively addressed in 1979. Racial minorities were found to have almost twice the infant mortality of whites, a higher proportion of maternity-related and other reproductive health problems, and the highest incidence of acute conditions among lowest-income females (U.S. Department of Health, Education, and Welfare, 1979, pp. 6-7). Minorities and low-income groups had higher death rates than the general population for four of the five leading causes of death: heart disease, cancer, stroke and diabetes. These reports, however, provided only limited information on the specific health needs of women.

The two most recent government reports on racial/ethnic minorities are *Black and Minority Health* (USDHHS 1985a) and

Women's Health (USDHHS, 1985b). Several areas were identified as common to all of the groups and as contributing to poorer health status:

1. Ethnic minority women experience higher infant mortality rates, higher neonatal death rates and higher post-neonatal death rates. Low birthweight, which accounts for 60% of infant deaths, is higher among racial/ethnic minorities, especially Black women (12.4%) and Puerto Ricans (9.1%).
2. There is a greater prevalence of some chronic diseases among racial/ethnic minority women, such as diabetes, hypertension, cardiovascular diseases, and certain types of cancer such as cervical cancer.
3. There is a lower life expectancy of five to seven years among racial/ethnic women than among their white counterparts, attributable to higher rates of chronic disease and less access to medical care systems, particularly for early detection and prevention of disease (USDHHS, 1985a).

In general, there is now a consensus among researchers that poor and racial/ethnic women are at a disadvantage in terms of their health status (e.g., Institute of Medicine, 1985). Overall assessments of the nature and types of disease patterns among the populations with respect to poor Black, Puerto Rican and Mexican-American women and immigrant women are available. The difficulty, however, lies in assessing health problems among different racial and ethnic subgroups, especially poor Caucasian women and women of racial/ethnic minority backgrounds because of the failure to control for the socioeconomic status and other quality-of-life indicators of the groups under study (see for example Camasso & Camasso, 1986). The changing composition of the family and the increasing numbers of employed women heads of households, with the anticipated adverse effect on their health status, make such information even more vital.

Of course, the health needs of low-income women are not necessarily distinct from her higher-income racial or ethnic peers, but the combination of her disadvantages of gender, class and racial/ethnic status increases the likelihood that she will have serious health needs and the probable likelihood that those needs will not be adequately met. Finally, although national health statistics are increasingly being compiled and reported by ethnicity, race and gender, local health statistics generally are not. Most hospitals and health service agencies usually do not systematically report health information by ethnicity or class background. Without such basic data on health status and health-seeking behavior among these populations, in-depth study and analysis of local trends are seriously limited.

The methodological limitations of the studies which have been conducted are most clearly illustrated in the area of reproductive health. Two areas of particular concern are adolescent mothers and women of childbearing age. Although our knowledge has increased in the areas of adolescent childbearing and maternal and child health, there are still many gaps with reference to poor and racial/ethnic minority women.

ADOLESCENT CHILDBEARING

Over the past twenty years a national decline in fertility levels has characterized a broad range of social groups within the United States, including women at all socioeconomic levels, racial/ethnic backgrounds and religious groups (Gibson, 1976; Rindfuss & Sweet, 1978). In contrast, the number of pregnancies and births among unmarried adolescent girls has greatly increased. The percentage of teen pregnancies has risen over the last ten years from 8.5% of 15- to 19-year-olds in 1971 to 16.2% in 1979. In their study of sexually active teenage girls, Zelnik and Kanter (1980) found an increase of 50% among those who had never used contraceptives. The percentage of unwed births within the adolescent population has risen 60% since 1965 and 300% since 1942 (Bolton, 1982; Zelnik, Kanter & Ford, 1981).

Teenage pregnancy and childbearing are now viewed as significant problems with negative psychological, social, medical, educational and economic impact. Adolescent pregnancy and parenthood have been found to carry a high risk of adverse consequences, both short- and long-term, for mother, child and family, leading Furstenburg (1976) to label it a "syndrome of defeat." Pregnant adolescents have been found to be obstetrically at risk, with maternal and infant mortality higher among teen mothers than among other groups. Nonfatal health complications have been found to be more common for teen mothers than for the population at large as well. Adolescent mothers are less likely to finish high school than other adolescents, which, combined with lack of childcare, severely limits occupational opportunities (Guttmacher, 1981).

With few exceptions, empirical research on adolescent sexuality and pregnancy has focused on Black and Anglo populations. Black adolescents were found to be more likely than Anglos to have nonmarital coitus without use of contraception, more likely to become pregnant and more likely to keep their babies (Zelnik, Kantner & Ford, 1981). Early inquiries have focused on the negative outcomes, and have relied on explanations based only on race and socioeconomic background. Not until the late 1970s was attention focused more extensively on the nature of the problem (e.g., socioeconomic antecedents), consequences and intervention strategies. Even now, however, the national concern with adolescent reproductive behavior has almost totally neglected the large Latino population, an exception being the recent work by Becerra and de Anda (1984).

Latinos are one of the fastest-growing ethnic groups in the United States. Research indicates that they will become the largest racial-ethnic minority group in the country during the first decade of the 21st century (Hayes-Bautista et al., 1986). Almost half of the Mexican-Americans, who make up 60% of the Latino population, are under 20 years of age (U.S. Bureau of the Census, 1984). For many years Latinos have had the highest fertility rate of any group identified in census data (Ventura & Heuser, 1981). The 1980 statistics show that a relatively large proportion, nearly one in five, of Latino births are to teenagers (Ventura, 1982). Although interest in and use of contraceptives by Latinas have been reported in some studies to be high, unmarried Latina adolescents have far fewer rates of contraceptive use than adolescents from other ethnic groups (Becerra & de Anda, 1984; Rochat et al., 1981; Stein, 1985; U.S. Department of Health, Education and Welfare, 1979).

Adolescent sexuality and fertility behavior are influenced by experiences within the family, peer group, school, media and other institutions. Historical background, sociocultural values and norms, socioeconomic status, ethnicity and religion have all been found to contribute to the development and expression of adolescent sexuality (Chilman, 1983). These are critical social variables that suggest an interactive model of developmental, cultural and environmental forces that affects adolescent decision-making and behaviors. This perspective suggests that relevant directions for the prevention of the "syndrome of defeat" associated with adolescent childbearing may be found. In conducting research that is sensitive to this constellation of factors, women's strengths in their sexual decision-making also may be more fully appreciated.

MATERNAL AND CHILD HEALTH

There is important evidence that points to ethnic variation in pregnancy outcomes for mothers and infants, with Black and Latina women placed at higher risk than women in most other ethnic groups. Mexican-American women between the ages of 15-29 have a higher percentage of deaths from complications of pregnancy than Anglos (U.S. Subcommittee on Census and Population, 1983). Birth weights are 2.3 times lower for babies born to Black women in California than for Caucasians, and are also lower for Latinas (Medina, 1980; Williams, 1980). In a recent analysis of perinatal outcomes among Medicaid recipients in California, Norris and Williams (1984, pp. 1113-1114) found that white non-Hispanic women had the highest absolute and proportional decreases in the percentage of low-weight (less than 2500 grams) births, while Blacks had the lowest decrease. In 1978, nearly 80% of Caucasian mothers began prenatal care in the first trimester compared with 60% of Black mothers (Health U.S. 1981, p. 12). National data are not readily available for Latinas. Nevertheless, Medina (1980), in his study of Latina reproductive health in California, found that in 1976 almost twice as many Latinas as Caucasians or Blacks had late or no prenatal care.

Several investigators have noted the relationship between late or no prenatal care and poorer pregnancy outcomes (Boone, 1982; Jackson, 1981; Medina, 1980; Norris & Williams, 1984; Showstack, Budetti & Minkler, 1984). All of these authors also suggest that research and development of reasonable solutions and interventions are needed to improve maternal and child health. Despite these recommendations, there remains a significant gap in the maternal and child health literature for poor and racial/ethnic groups, and particularly around factors of class and ethnicity as they affect utilization of prenatal care.

In the last decade, two major questions have guided the study of prenatal care and outcome: the aspects of care that make a difference and the characteristics of the populations who seek care. The mechanisms whereby the mother's emotional state influences progress during the pregnancy and course of delivery are not known. Some studies, however, have identified nonmedical factors such as education, social support and improved nutrition as contributing to more positive pregnancy outcomes (Barnard & Sumner, 1981, pp. 62-64). Differences in birth outcomes among different racial/ethnic groups seem to be related to social class and to lack of early initiation of prenatal care or no prenatal care (Boone, 1982; Jackson, 1981; Medina, 1980; Norris & Williams, 1984; Showstack et al., 1984). At present, little information is available on factors that contribute to the late initiation of prenatal care, either within racial/ethnic groups or between groups.

Maternal and child well-being are also influenced by psychosocial factors such as chronic stress and social support, and by breastfeeding practices, which are in turn reflective of social factors. Life stress has been examined as a factor in obstetrical complications. Gorsuch and Key (1974) found that major life events occurring six months prior to the pregnancy or during the second and third trimesters were associated with abnormalities. Social support has been shown to be an important factor in the maintenance of well-being and in decisions regarding help-seeking behaviors (Dohrenwend & Dohrenwend, 1978). Research on social support and health more broadly strengthens the evidence that support may be an important factor in pregnancy, labor, delivery, and prematurity (Cobb, 1976; Gottlieb, 1981; Heller, 1979;

House, 1981; Wallston, Alagna, DeVellis & DeVellis, 1981).
Nuckolls, Cassell and Caplan (1972) found that women with
high life change and low psychosocial assets (i.e., social support, positive attitudes towards pregnancy) suffered more complications at delivery than women with more assets or fewer life
changes. Similarly, Lewis and Jones (1980) found that adolescents who had high stress and low social support also had more
problems in delivery than other groups with stronger social support or less stress.

Race, ethnicity and class may be discriminators of breastfeeding behavior, which is considered an important factor in both the
physical and emotional development of the infant (Jelliffe & Jeliffe, 1982). In recent years, breastfeeding behavior has become
more common among well-educated, high-socioeconomic status
women, particularly Caucasians, than among lower-income
women, particularly Latinas and Blacks. In part, this phenomenon is related to education, participation in childbirth education
and a supportive family and institutional environment. Many
middle-class women now select physicians and birth settings
based on compatible values, such as environments supportive of
breastfeeding. In a recent review of the literature on breastfeeding, Scrimshaw and colleagues (1984) conclude that very little
empirical evidence is available on the factors influencing low-
income Black and Latina women in their infant feeding decisions. Furthermore, Scrimshaw, Engle and Horseley's (1985)
work with Mexican-American women in Los Angeles identified
institutional barriers to breastfeeding, particularly in the hospital
of delivery. Molina (1983, p. 39) states that breastfeeding behavior requires active encouragement among Latina women, who
tend to rely on bottle formulas because they believe this method
is more nourishing. The need "to identify and reduce barriers
which keep women from beginning or continuing to breastfeed
their infants" was also noted by the U.S. Surgeon General, as
was the need to encourage such breastfeeding in the Latina and
Black population as a whole (USDHSS, 1984).

To date, few studies have examined the importance of social
class as a variable, and the most recent work in the field of childbirth has minimized this factor (Nelson, 1982, p. 3509). Accord-

ing to Nelson (1982), the majority of studies in reproductive health have been conducted on Anglo middle-class women who have education, knowledge and familiarity with the health care system. Nelson also concludes with the precaution that a study that ignores social class as a variable may well lead to unsound generalizations.

THE CONTEXT OF HEALTH STATUS
AND FUNCTIONING

The low-income woman has basic primary and preventive health needs for herself and her family. She must address these needs using a male-dominated, affluent health care delivery system oriented toward tertiary care. At each step of the way the woman is faced with complex responsibilities and encounters multiple barriers, while being responsible for maintaining wellness and preventing illness for her family under socioeconomic conditions that promote mental and physical illness. She must sort out those health concerns that are most appropriately alleviated through traditional support, such as information and assistance from family and community, and those that are best served by modern medicine and institutional providers. She must learn how the health care system is organized, where to seek appropriate care, and how to linguistically and culturally translate their concerns into information that will be meaningful to health professionals. She bears the burden of evaluating prescribed treatment, both in terms of modern medical risk and in terms of congruence with her own culture and life-style. At the same time, poor and racial/ethnic women are most likely to be heads of households, to have larger families, to bear the heaviest burden of caring for the health and well-being of all family members, to be in the poorest health themselves, to experience the greatest psychologically induced symptoms or illnesses, and to be at highest medical risk, particularly during pregnancy and childbirth (Hurst & Zambrana, 1980; Marieskind, 1980, pp. 35-36; USDHHS, 1985a).

Racial/ethnic women share a disproportionately large responsibility not only for the care and nurturing of the children but also for their support. This responsibility is particularly striking given

the increase in families headed by women and their disproportionate stratification in the labor force. A study of single parents
found that poor health, personal illness or the illness of a child
or relative prevented a number of respondents from entering the
labor market (Morgan, 1981). Hurst and Zambrana (1980) also
found that poor health, particularly after childbirth, was a major
factor in accounting for the discontinuous work histories among
Puerto Rican women in New York.

Understanding access issues among poor and minority women
requires consideration of economic, cultural and systemic factors
(Dutton, 1978). While middle-class women are at least able to
enter the health care system via a personal physician who can act
as buffer, link, and translator, poor women confront impersonal
institutions on their own. Minority women, particularly Hispanics, may also be handicapped by language, in addition to lack of
education, information and insurance.

Insurance coverage is a major barrier. Black and Puerto Ricans
were twice as likely as whites not to have health insurance.
Among Mexican-Americans the noninsured rate is three and one-
half times greater than that of white non-Hispanics. Individuals
with low family income were found to be less likely to have
health insurance. The most frequent reason cited for lack of
health insurance reported by all racial/ethnic groups was inability
to pay. Among Mexican-Americans, low rates of insurance coverage may also be accounted for by employers who generally do
not provide such coverage as an employment benefit (Trevino &
Moss, 1983).

While increasing numbers of studies point to a relationship
between health status and social roles, class and cultural variables as causal factors remain a poorly understood aspect of the
health of low-income and minority women. Although cultural
practices of Hispanic groups are related to family life and beliefs
in nontraditional sources of health care, class and institutional
barriers may be stronger predictors of health care-seeking behavior and health status (Chesney et al., 1982). As is true in many
areas, the existence of cultural determinants of health behaviors
tend to vary inversely with social-class standing.

Language and educational barriers prevent the poor, Hispanic
and minority woman from receiving most of the public health

education that the middle class now takes for granted. She is not exposed to the controversies surrounding unnecessary surgery, informed consent, and sterilization reported regularly in the English-language press, which would make her a more discerning health "consumer." She has limited access to evaluations of potentially dangerous products conducted by such consumer organizations as the Consumer's Union or by the Food and Drug Administration. Books about family care, female health-related concerns, or how to be an active health consumer are rarely translated to Spanish and, even when they are, the information is not accessible to women who have little formal education, money or exposure to bookstores and libraries.

While studies of the health needs of poor and racial/ethnic women are important, it is most critical that these studies be sensitive to historical, cultural and socioeconomic factors. Poor women have been subjected to persistent degrading treatment by the medical care system (Corea, 1977; Scully, 1973; Shaw, 1974). Researchers need to become aware of the situational factors that affect poor and minority women's health care status to avoid the perpetuation of stereotypes and nonconstructive labelling.

A MODEL FOR UNDERSTANDING THEIR HEALTH NEEDS

Data and a research agenda would be meaningless without a context in which to interpret it (Becerra & Zambrana, 1985). Thus the health status of poor and minority women should be understood in relation to their race, class and gender. Existing models and analyses can only provide limited explanatory power if directly applied to poor and racial/ethnic populations. For example, the analytic frameworks that have been developed, such as Becker's (1974) Health Belief Model and Aday and colleagues' (1980) Access to Care Model, have emerged from the study of dominant-culture middle-class populations. In a recent review by Verbrugge (1986) on gender and health, the author fails to address differential risks among women due to race and class.

A model that seeks to interpret data on these groups in a meaningful way must expand its parameters to take into account clearly defined socioeconomic, racial, cultural, and regional variables that have a particular relationship with access to health care resources, and psychosocial variables that address the relationship between health status and functioning, chronic life stress, sources of social support, work status and occupational history. It has been suggested that the "mere struggle to provide for one's family causes half of all Black female adults to live in psychological stress" (*Health Factsheet of Black Women*, Winter, 1983). Occupational history may also be an important determinant of the health status of poor and racial/ethnic women who work (Mullings, 1984). Black women have a 39% greater chance of sustaining job-related disease and serious work-related injuries than nonminorities. Hispanics are overrepresented in such high-risk industries as construction, garment industry and metal mining (USDHHS, 1985, pp. 52-54).

The ethnic and class differences within racial/ethnic groups must be carefully controlled for. A number of researchers have argued that heterogeneity within Hispanic and Black groups by both class and country of origin must be recognized, particularly among the Hispanic population, which varies along the three parameters of race, ethnicity and class. Data on Hispanics must be analyzed by region and cultural background (e.g., Puerto Rican, Mexican-American and Cuban). Socio-demographic characteristics among these subgroups will also vary, together with health indicators. For individuals of Hispanic origin, the concept of acculturation needs close evaluation. In this author's opinion, the measurement of acculturation is a proxy for social class, which must be understood within the context both of the recency of arrival (if an immigrant) and of language proficiency as a measure of an individual's familiarity with dominant-culture systems. One recent study found that low acculturation was highly correlated with low social class and lower use of health services (Chesney et al., 1982).

This interactive model requires that social, behavioral and environmental variables be clearly defined and examined both in designing studies and in interpreting data on poor and racial/ethnic populations (see, for example, Carr & Wolfe, 1979). Dill

(1983) has aptly stated the importance of a more comprehensive perspective on racial/ethnic women:

> Concretely, and from a research perspective this suggests the importance of looking at both the structures which shape women's lives and their self-presentations. This would provide us not only with a means of gaining insight into the ways in which racial, class and sexual oppression are viewed but with a means of generating conceptual categories that will aid us in extending our knowledge of their situation. At the same time, this new knowledge will broaden and even reform our conceptualization of women's situation.

A RESEARCH AGENDA: BEGINNING DIRECTIONS FOR FUTURE RESEARCH

The recognition that poor and minority female populations have special needs is not a novel idea. Many of the initial public health endeavors in the late 19th and early 20th centuries, such as milk stations and neighborhood health centers, were aimed at women and children. Endeavors in the 1960s such as the "War on Poverty" programs were also geared to services for poor and minority women and their families (Davis & Schoen, 1978).

This section proposes a selective research agenda in the areas of reproductive health, health practices and cancer, poor and racial/ethnic minority women and aging, and the relationship between chronic life stress, social support and health status and functioning. It should be recognized, however, that there are many other areas in which significant gaps in knowledge severely limit our understanding of minority health needs. For example, one rapidly escalating public health problem is the incidence of AIDS among minority women and children. It has been shown that increasing numbers of new pediatric AIDS cases are among Hispanic and Black children. The agenda is proposed within the context of a model that recognizes the plurality and interactive nature of factors influencing health status.

Reproductive Health

Reproductive health represents a critical area of health care for poor and minority women because it includes those aspects of reproduction currently subject to public legislation and political action. Abortion, sterilization and contraception are issues important to all women, but in many ways policy and practice, coupled with historic class and race inequalities, have made these particularly significant subjects for minority women, who have the least knowledge and are the most vulnerable population groups. A number of critical research areas that require attention are the relationship between occupational hazards and reproductive outcome; the prevalence of Caesarian section and hysterectomy; studies on the effects and context of materials presented in family life/sex education classes in schools; efficacy of informed consent procedures currently in use (with comparisons of experiences of different ethnic and social groups); studies of providers and recipients of genetic counseling; and amniocentesis and women of color.[5]

Health Practices and Cancer

An important area of investigation includes health practices such as nutrition, substance use, and exercise, and their relationship to socioeconomic status and influence on health status and functioning. Mounting evidence suggests that poor health practices, or behavioral risks among lower-socioeconomic groups, may contribute to their higher health risks. A number of studies have shown a relationship between health practices, ethnicity and social class (Hamburg et al., 1982; Marcus & Crane, 1985). These preliminary findings need further investigation, using larger samples and including questions about drinking and smoking practices among poor and racial/ethnic women. Does lower use of alcohol and nicotine among Latina women contribute to more favorable birth outcomes, for example?

Major risk factors such as use of alcohol and tobacco, nutritional and dietary factors, and occupation are thought to account for approximately 72% of cancer mortality and 69% of incidence. Socioeconomic status also has been correlated with poorer survival from cancer and increased incidence of lung,

breast and cervical cancers among poor and minority women
(USDHHS, 1985a, pp. 87-97). Again, there is limited information on poor and minority women, especially Hispanic women.

In response to the lack of data on Hispanics, the National Cancer Institute (NCI), Division of Cancer Prevention and Control
has developed a Hispanic Cancer Control Program (HCCP). In
the last year the HCCP has completed an annotated bibliography
of literature on cancer and Hispanics (NCI, 1986a, 1986b). A
research agenda developed by NCI in April, 1986 defined the
need for the collection of data locally and nationally using ethnic
identifiers to develop cancer control interventions that address
inter-ethnic differences in cancer incidence, mortality and survival; and to conduct research that examines basic risk factors in
relationship to cancer incidence (NCI, 1986c), all virtually unex-
plored areas.

Aging of Poor and Racial/Ethnic Women

There is a dearth of information about aging in the racial/eth-
nic subgroup although it is known that these women become
poorer earlier and at a greater rate. Understanding the qualitative
experiences of these women will require investigating their labor
market experiences, the types and nature of benefits accrued over
time, if any, and the influence of their work experiences on their
health status. The subjective meaning of aging among the different cohorts of poor and racial/ethnic women is also an important
issue. Exploration of the meaning and quality of aging necessi-
tates examining their educational and work backgrounds and
whether these contribute to a sense of life satisfaction. The economic and social options open to these women after rearing their
families, particularly if they are divorced or widowed and have
not had continuous work participation outside the home, are
other issues.

Chronic Life Stress and Health Status and Functioning

The inquiry into stress must assess the nature and extent of
chronic stress over time and its impact on health status and functioning. It must conceptualize stress in relation to the quality of
life issues of being poor, female and of color (see, for example,

Vega & Mirande, 1985). Analysis of social support, a buffering factor in most stress models, is often fraught with methodological difficulties and rarely focuses on poor and minority women. In a recent review, Vaux (1985:89) emphasizes the lack of comparative research on social support and how "relatively little is known about how it varies across subgroups in the population." Refinement of these conceptual areas and cross-validation of instruments to assure that they indeed measure these concepts for poor and racial/ethnic women needs research. One important direction may be to explore the relationship between nature and types of stress, sources of social support, and chronic illness. In a cross-cultural study, it would be important to examine the differential impact of these variables on the various groups.

IMPLEMENTING THE AGENDA

Formulation of a model and a research agenda for poor and racial/ethnic women is an important step toward achieving the goal of improved quality of life for low-income and racial/ethnic individuals. The issues and agenda developed in the several reports and policy statements discussed here clearly point in the same direction. Given such agreement on issues and agenda, an equally significant question arises: Who is responsible for seeking further understanding of the problems and for proposing and implementing policy solutions that are both relevant and appropriate?

The answer to this question is both simple and complex. It is simple in that the major health care needs of poor and racial/ethnic populations are generally known, namely, better preventive and primary health care services. The major issue for poor and racial/ethnic populations, especially the women, is access and availability of services. It is also complex in that the link between needs identification, policy formulation and the development of social welfare programs is problematic at best. An example is the move for cost-containment in medical care that has led to the closure, defunding and underfunding of public health facilities and to decreases in medical care benefits for the indigent. Thus, whatever the merits of the economic debate, the already underserved segment of the population is accumulating the disadvantages of increased health care costs and reduced services. In this author's opinion, a solution is to develop and implement a national health insurance program geared to respond to identified needs (Physicians' Forum, 1985) and to provide services to local communities, with community-level research supported as an integral part of all community-based health care services. This will assure the on-going assessment of needs as the basis for future social welfare policy formulation and planning. The preeminent need is to lower the barriers that continue to limit access of the poor and of racial/ethnic populations to essential human services.

NOTES

1.Throughout this article, the terms "women of color," "minority women" and "racial/ethnic women" are used interchangeably.

2.There are very limited data on low-income white women. National data are aggregated by White, Black and Other, and therefore do not reflect class distinctions.

3.The major focus of data presented will be in reference to Black, Mexican-American and Puerto Rican subgroups. These are the largest racial/ethnic minority groups in the U.S. However, it is recognized that other recent-immigrant groups from the Carribean and Central America are at an economic disadvantage and have special health needs. The estimates of the number of undocumented workers in the U.S. range from 3 million to 12 million. Native Americans and Asian groups also represent distinct racial/ethnic populations and share a number of common conditions that contribute to poorer health status.

4.There is tremendous diversity among and within the Hispanic population. This diversity is related in part to class position, cultural differences based on country of origin, generational differences in the U.S., and regional/geographic distribution. Generalizations based on national data must be made with caution and understanding of the domains of diversity.

5.A detailed research agenda has been developed by the Women's Rights Litigation Clinic and the Institute for Research on Women at Rutgers University in their project on "Reproductive Laws for the 1990s." The major areas identified are: social, economic and technical aspects of infertility; use of reproductive services; and protections for choice and prenatal screening. The research agenda calls for a particular focus on how these issues affect women of color.

REFERENCES

Aday, L. A., Andersen, R. & Fleming, G. V. (1980). *Health care in the U.S.: Equitable for Whom?* Beverly Hills, CA: Sage Publications.

Andrade, S. J. (1982). Family roles of Hispanic women: Stereotypes, empirical findings and implications for research. In R.E. Zambrana (Ed.), *Latina women in transition*. New York: Fordham University, Hispanic Research Center.

Andrade, S. J. (Ed.) (1983). *Latino families in the United States: A resourcebook for family education*. Education Department, Planned Parenthood Federation of America.

Baca-Zinn, M. (1982). Review essay: Mexican-American women in the social sciences. *Signs, 8* (Winter), 259-272.

Barnard, K. E. & Sumner, G. A. (1981). The health of women with fertility-related needs. In L.V. Klerman (Ed.), *Research priorities in maternal and child health: Report of a conference June 9-10, 1981*. Office of Maternal and Child Health, HSA, PHS, U.S. Department of Health and Human Services.

Becerra, R. M. & Zambrana, R. E. (1985). Methodological approaches to research on Hispanics. *Social Work Research and Abstracts, 21* (2) (Summer), 42-49.

Becerra, R. M. & deAnda, D. (1984). Pregnancy and motherhood among Mexican American adolescents. *Health and Social Work, 9,*(2), 106-123.

Becker, M. H. (1974). *The health belief model and personal health behavior*. NJ: Charles B. Slack, Inc.

Bolton, F. G. (1982). *The pregnant adolescent: Problems of premature parenthood*. Beverly Hills, CA: Sage Publications.

Boone, M. S. (1982). A socio-medical study of infant mortality among disadvantaged Blacks. *Human organization, 41* (3).

Camasso, M. J. & Camasso, A. E. (1986). Social supports, undesirable life events and psychological distress in a disadvantaged population. *Social Service Review*, September, 378-394.

Carr, W. & Wolfe, S. (1979). Unmet needs as sociomedical indicators. In J. Elinson, & A. Siegmann (Eds.), *Sociomedical health indicators*. Farmingdale, NY: Baywood.

Chesney, A. P., Chavira, J. A., Hall, R. P. & Gary, H. E. Jr. (1982). Barriers to medical care of Mexican-Americans: The role of social class, acculturation, and social isolation. *Medical Care, 20* (9), 883-891.

Chilman, C. (1983). *Adolescent sexuality in a changing American society*. New York: John Wiley and Sons.

Cobb, S. (1976). Social support as a moderator of life stress. *Psychosomatic Medicine, 38* (5), 300-314.

Corea, G. (1977). *The hidden malpractice: How American medicine treats women as patients and professionals*. New York: William Morrow.

Davis, K. & Schoen, C. (1978). *Health and the war on poverty: A ten-year appraisal*. Washington, DC: Brookings.

Dill, B. T. (1983). Race, class and gender: Prospects for an all-inclusive sisterhood. *Feminist Studies, 9* (Spring), 131-150.

Dohrenwend, D. B. & Dohrenwend, B. P. (1978). Some issues in research on stressful life events. *Journal of Nervous and Mental Disorders, 166*, 7-15.

Dutton, D. B. (1978). Explaining the low use of health services by the poor: Costs, attitudes or delivery systems? *American Sociological Review, 43*, 348-368.

Furstenburg, F. F. (1976). *Unplanned parenthood: The social consequences of teenage childbearing*. New York: Free Press.

Gibson, C. (1976). THe U.S. fertility decline, 1961-1975: The contribution of changes in marital status and marital fertility. *Family Planning Perspectives, 8*, 249-252.

Gorsuch, R. L. & Key, M. K. (1974). Abnormalities of pregnancy as a function of anxiety and life stress. *Psychosomatic Medicine, 36*, 352-361.

Guttmacher Institute (1981). *Teenage pregnancy: The problem hasn't gone away*. New York: Alan Guttmacher Institute.

Jeliffe, D. B. & Jeliffe, E. F. P. (1982). Cultural traditions and nutritional practices related to pregnancy and lactation. *Symposium Swedish Nutritional Foundation*, 48-61.

Hamburg, D. A., Elliot, G. R. & Parron, D. L. (1982). *Health and behavior frontiers of research in the biobehavioral sciences.* Institute of Medicine. Washington, D.C.: National Academy Press.

Hayes-Bautista D. E., Schink, W. O. & Chapa, J. (1986). *The burden of support: The young Latino population in an aging American society.* Palo Alto, CA: Stanford University Press.

Health factsheet on Black women (1983, winter). National Women's Health Project, National Women's Health Network.

Heller, K. (1979). The effect of social support: prevention of treatment implications. In A. P. Goldstein & F. H. Kanfer (Eds.), *Maximizing treatment gains in transfer enhancement in psychotherapy.* New York: Academic Press.

House, J. S. (1981). *Work, stress and social support.* Reading, MA: Addison-Wesley Publishing Co.

Hurst, M. & Zambrana, R. E. (1980). The health careers of urban women: a study in East Harlem. *Signs 5* (3), part 2, 112-126. (Reprinted in C. R. Stimpson, E. Dixler, M. J. Nelson, & K. B. Jatrakis [eds.], *Women and the American cities.* Chicago: University of Chicago Press, 1980, 109-123.)

Institute of Medicine, Division of Health Promotion and Disease Prevention (1985, January). *The prevention of low birthweight.* Washington, DC: National Academy Press.

Jackson, J. J. (1981). Urban Black Americans. In A. Harwood (Ed.), *Ethnicity and medical care.* Cambridge, MA: Harvard University Press.

Kanter, R. (1977). *Work and family in the United States: A critical review and agenda for research and policy.* New York: Russell Sage Foundation.

Lewis, J. D. & Jones, A. C. (1980). Psychological stress, social support systems and pregnancy complications in adolescents. Paper presented at the Annual Meetings of the American Psychological Association, Montreal.

Marcus, A. C. & Crance, L. A. (1985). Smoking behavior among U.S. Latinos: An emerging challenge for public health. *American Journal of Public Health, 75* (2), 169-172.

Marieskind, H. I. (1980). *Women in the health system.* St. Louis: C. V. Mosby.

Massey, D. (1982, March). The demographic and economic position of Hispanics in the United States: 1980. Report to the National Commission for Employment Policy.

McAdoo, H. & Pearce, D. (1981). *Women and children: Alone and in poverty.* Washington, DC: U.S. Government Printing Office.

Medina, A. S. (1979, September). Hispanic reproductive health in California, 1976-1977. Paper presented at the Hispanic Health Services Research Conference, sponsored by the National Center for Health Services Research at the University of New Mexico, Albuquerque, Institute for Applied Research Services.

Molina, C. (1983). Family health promotion: A conceptual framework for "La Salud" and "El Bienestar" in Latino communities. In S. J. Andrade (Ed.), *Latino families in the United States: A resourcebook for family life education.* New York: Education Department, Planned Parenthood Federation of America.

Moore, E. (1980). Women and health: United States. *Public Health Reports,* September-October supplement.

Morgan, L.A. (1981, August). *Access to training programs: Barriers encountered by Hispanic female heads-of-household in New York City.* New York: Puerto Rican Legal Defense and Education Fund.

Muller, C. (1979). Women and health statistics. *Women and Health, 4* (1), 37-59.

Mullings, L. (1984). Minority women, work and health, In W. Chavkin (Ed.), *Double exposure: Women's health hazards on the job and at home.* New York: Monthly Review Press.

Nathanson, C. A. (1980). Social roles and health status among women: The significance of employment. *Social Science and Medicine, 14*A, 463-471.

National Cancer Institute (1986a). *Annotated bibliography of the literature on cancer in Hispanics.* Rockville, MD: NCI, Division of Cancer Prevention and Control, Hispanic Cancer Control Program.

———— (1986b). *Information systems and data sources related to surveillance indicators for monitoring the progress of Hispanics toward achieving the cancer control national objectives.* Rockville, MD: NCI, Division of Cancer Prevention and Control, Hispanic Cancer Control Program.

———— (1986c). *Proceedings summary of the Hispanic cancer control program workshop.* (April 17-18). Rockville, MD: NCI, Division of Cancer Prevention and Control, Hispanic Cancer Control Program.

Navarro, V. (Ed.) (1977). *Health and medical care in the U.S.: A critical analysis.* New York: Baywood.

Nelson, M. K. (Ed.) (1982). The effect of childbirth preparation on women of different social classes. *Journal of Health and Social Behavior, 23* (4), 339-352.

Norris, F. D. & Williams, R. (1984). Perinatal outcomes among Medicaid recipients in California. *American Journal of Public Health, 74* (10).

Nuckolls, K. B., Cassel, J. & Kaplan, B. H. (1972). Psychosocial assets, life crises, and the prognosis of pregnancy. *American Journal of Epidemiology, 95*, 431-441.

Olesen, V. (Ed.) (1977). *Women and their health: Research implications for a new era.* Springfield, VA: National Technical Information Service.

Physicians' Forum (1986). A proposal for a national health policy. *Monday Comments, 28*, February 3.

Rindfuss, R. & Sweet, J. (1978). The pervasiveness of postwar fertility trends in the United States. In K. Taeuber, L. Bumpas & J. Sweet (Eds.), *Social demography.*

Rochat, R. (1981). Family planning practices among Anglo and Hispanic women in the U.S. counties bordering Mexico. *Family Planning Perspectives, 13*, 176-180.

Scrimshaw, S. C. M., Engle, P. L. & Horseley, K. (1985). Use of prenatal services by women of Mexican origin and descent in Los Angeles. *Prevention in Human Services*, Spring.

Scrimshaw, S. C. M. Engle, P. L., Arnold, A. & Haynes, K. (1984). The cultural context of breastfeeding in the United States. Paper presented at the Surgeon General's Workshop on Breastfeeding and Human Lactation, Rochester, New York. Summarized in the *Report of the Surgeon General's Workshop on Breastfeeding and Human Lactation*, U.S. Department of Health and Human Services, DHHS Publication No. HRS-D-MC, 84-2 (1984a).

Scully, D. (1980). *Men who control women's health.* Boston: Houghton Mifflin.

Shaw, N. S. (1974). *Forced labor: Maternity care in the U.S.* New York: Pergamon Press.

Showstack, J. A., Budetti, P. P. & Minkler, D. (1984). Factors associated with birthweight: An exploration of the roles of prenatal care and length of gestation. *American Journal of Public Health, 74* (9), 1003-1008.

Stein, S. J. (1985). Factors related to contraceptive use among Mexican-American adolescents. Doctoral Dissertation, Wright Institute, Los Angeles.

Trevino, F. M. & Mass, A. J. (1983). Health insurance coverage and physician visits among Hispanic and non-Hispanic people. In *Health: United States, 1983.* Washington, DC: U.S. Public Health Service, National Center for Health Statistics, DHHS Publication No. (PHS) 84-1232.

Trevino, F. M. & Mass, A. J. (1984). Health insurance for Hispanic, Black and White Americans. *Vital and Health Statistics.* Series 10, No. 148. Washington, DC: U.S. Public Health Service, National Center for Health Statistics, DHHS Publication No. (PHS) 84-1576.

Trevino, F. M. (1986, April). Cross-cultural differences in health insurance coverage and access to medical care. Paper presented to Congressional Women's Caucus, Congressional Black Caucus, and Congressional Hispanic Caucus.

U.S. Bureau of the Census (1984, July). *Population division.* Washington, DC: U.S. Government Printing Office.

U.S. Commission on Civil Rights (1982). *Unemployment and underemployment among Blacks, Hispanics and women.* Washington, DC: Government Printing Office.

U.S. Department of Health and Human Services (1981). *Health: United States 1981.* Hyattsville, MD: U.S. Public Health Service, Publication No. (PHS) 82-1232.

U.S. Department of Health, Education and Welfare (1979). (Rudov, M. & Santangelo, N., preparers.) *Health status of low-income groups.* Washington, DC: U.S. Government Printing Office. DHEW Publication No. (HRA) 79-627.

U.S. Department of Health and Human Services (1984). Report of the Surgeon General's workshop on breastfeeding and human lactation. DHHS Publication No. HRS-D-MC 84-2.

U.S. Department of Health and Human Services (1985a). *Black and Minority Health.* Report of the Secretary's Task Force, Executive Summary, Vol.1.

U.S. Department of Health and Human Services (1985b). *Women's Health.* Report of the Public Health Service Task Force on Women's Health Issues (Vol. II), Washington, DC.

U.S. Subcommittee on Census and Population (1983). *The Hispanic population of the U.S.: An overview.* Washington, DC: U.S. Government Printing Office.

Vaux, A. (1985). Variations in social support associated with gender, ethnicity and age. *Journal of Social Issues, 41* (1), 89-110.

Vega, W. M. & Miranda, M. R. (1985). *Stress and Hispanic mental health.* Washington, DC: US DHHS, National Institute of Mental Health.

Ventura, S. & Heuser, R. (1981). Births of Hispanic parentage, 1978. *Monthly Vital Statistics Report, 32* (supplement). Hyattsville, MD: National Center for Health Services Research, Public Health Service.

Verbrugge, L. M. (1985). Gender and health: An update on the hypotheses and evidence. *Journal of Health and Social Behavior, 26,* 156-182.

Wallston, B. S., Alagna, S. W., DeVellis, B. M. & Devellis, R. F. (in press). Support and physical health. *Health Psychology.*

Williams, R. (1980). Monitoring perinatal mortality rates: California, 1970 to 1976. *American Journal of Obstetrics and Gynecology, 136* (5), 559-568.

Zambrana, R. E. and Swanteson, E. (1979, November). Hispanic women as caretakers: Conflict or resolution? Paper presented at the Annual Meetings of the American Public Health Association, New York.

Zelnik, M. & Kantner, J. (1980). Sexual activity, contraceptive use and pregnancy among metropolitan area teenagers: 1971-1979. *Family Planning Perspectives, 12,* 230-237.

Zelnik, M., Kantner, J. & Ford, K. (1981). *Sex and pregnancy in adolescence.* Beverly Hills, CA: Sage Publications.

State-Level Public Policy
as a Predictor of
Individual and Family Well-Being

Shirley L. Zimmerman, PhD

SUMMARY. This exploratory study examines the relationship between state-level public policy and individual and family well-being and factors that affect it. The inquiry, based on exchange and choice theories, assumes that state-level public policy reflects states' awareness of the needs of individuals and families, their ability to predict the future in failing to meet them, and the extent to which the norm of reciprocity prevails in the 50 states. Measures of states' collective choices were states' per capita expenditures for public welfare, education, and health, and per capita taxes in 1980; measures of states' individual and well- or ill-being, or social malaise, were states' teenage birthrates, infant death rates, and suicide rates. Taken into account as antecedent and intervening variables were age, gender, and racial composition, income distribution, marital, socioeconomic, and employment status of states' populations, and attitudes toward public spending.

The findings show that *higher* state expenditures for public welfare and for education indeed contribute to individual and family well-being as measured by lower state rates of suicide and teenage births. States per capita spending for education, which together with state per capita spending for public welfare was a

Shirley L. Zimmerman is Associate Professor, Family Social Science, University of Minnesota, 290 McNeal Hall, 1985 Buford, St. Paul, MN 55108.

This research was made possible by the University of Minnesota, Agricultural Experiment Station, St. Paul, MN.

The author would like to thank the following persons for their interest in the research on which this manuscript is based and for their comments and suggestions relative to the manuscript itself: Edwin Shneidman, Phillips Cutright, Joseph Rothberg, and Barry Ensminger. The author alone is responsible for any errors in or misinterpretations of the study's finding.

positive predictor of school completion rates and positively associated with states' income level, accounted for almost all of the
variance in states' per capita taxes. State spending for public welfare was *not* a predictor of state per capita taxes.

These findings are cause for considerable concern given the
reduced role of the federal government in human affairs, particularly in states whose choices violate the assumptions underlying
exchange and choice theories and the norm of reciprocity which
says that people should help, not hurt, others.

This inquiry concerns itself with the relationship between
state-level public policy and individual and family well- or ill-
being, and factors that affect it. The period selected for the analysis, 1980 to 1982, is important because philosophically it represents a turning point in the history of the United States with
respect to the role of the federal government in human affairs.
The "New Federalism" and the budget cuts that accompanied it
signaled a dramatic change in federal-state relationships and in
the funding of many health and social service programs that
states administer with federal dollars (Knapp, 1982). Such cuts
occurred at a time when the economies of many states, particularly those in the Mid- and Northwest, were in serious trouble
because of changing technology, foreign competition, high interest rates, and high unemployment rates. In addition, many states,
having passed tax relief measures in the wake of the taxpayers'
revolt of the late 1970s, were left with diminished and diminishing financial reserves to fill the fiscal void created by the federal
budget cuts. At the same time, the New Federalism gave states
increased discretion with respect to the services they provide, for
whom, and under what conditions.

THE RESEARCH PERSPECTIVE

Exchange and choice theories (Ekeh, 1974; Levi-Strauss,
1969; Nye, 1979) provided the perspective that guided the research. From this perspective, state-level public policy is viewed
as collective choice (Olson, 1974) that reflects the adequacy and
accuracy of available information, the ability to predict the future
in terms of anticipated outcomes, and prevailing values relative

to the achievement of specified outcomes. According to exchange and choice theories, the value assigned to given outcomes determines whether they are regarded as costs or rewards. The assumption is that alternatives are chosen that promise the most favorable ratio of rewards to costs. However, avoidance of costs can be potentially costly because it can result in loss of rewards and in costly future outcomes. In this study, collective choice takes the form of state per capita expenditures for health, education, and social programs of various kinds as well as tax levies on individuals to meet the costs such programs entail. The assumption was that these choices reflect states' awareness of the needs of individuals and families and states' ability to predict and anticipate future costs in failing to meet them.

The choices also reflect the extent to which the norm of reciprocity prevails in the 50 states (Gouldner, 1960), taking into account states' fiscal capacities (Dye, 1975; Terrell, 1986); the demographics of their populations (Eulau & Eyestone, 1968); and prevailing ideology or values (Wilensky, 1975). In exchange theory, the norm of reciprocity takes precedence over the maximization of rewards relative to costs and is considered necessary for social life to continue. It implies that people should help, not hurt, others just as others should help, not hurt, them. The norm may be applied over time at both interpersonal and societal levels, those who have been helped by others in the past helping those who need help in the present, and those receiving help in the present helping those who may need help in the future.

Outcome Indicators of Collective Choice: Teenage Birthrates

Research has shown that social, psychological, cultural, physiological, and economic factors are all associated with adolescent pregnancy (Chilman, 1983; Cutright, 1972; Gottschalk et al., 1964). Adolescence begins around age 12 and generally ends at age 20. It is a period when identities are formed, bodily changes and adaptations to sexuality occur, experimentation with adult roles begin, and adult roles are assumed (Erickson, 1968; Piaget, 1967). Eager to be in control of their own lives, teenagers often rebel against parents and their values (Cohn & Friedman, 1975;

Kriepe, 1983). Some teens view pregnancy and parenthood as a means for achieving adult status and the autonomy and independence they perceive as accompanying it (Kriepe, 1983), many not realizing that more is involved to parenthood than childbearing. Many also do not have the cognitive skills needed to practice birth control responsibly, such skills not developing until mid-adolescence (Chilman, 1980; Dembo & Lundell, 1979). Among teens in dysfunctional families, early sexual activity may be a means for obtaining the affection they do not receive from their families. Females are particularly vulnerable in that they tend to view sexuality as a means of giving and receiving love (Cvetkovich & Grote, 1979, 1980), while boys are particularly susceptible to peer pressure, encouraged by an imaginary audience to demonstrate their sexual prowess by seeking sexual encounters.

Research also speaks to the role that poverty and discrimination play in teenage pregnancy. According to Moore and Burt (1982), socioeconomic and racial differences in sexual activity and the probability of pregnancy can be attributed in part to the differential opportunity structure of low-income and minority teenagers. Many poor teenagers who have low educational achievement aspirations not only tend to view motherhood as their only viable option, but many also do not understand reasons for delaying it. Forced into the labor force by the demands of early childbearing before they are adequately prepared, many are trapped into a lifetime of low-paying, low prestige jobs that offer little satisfaction (Baldwin, 1984) and few opportunities for upward mobility. Associated with teenage childbearing are early dependence; limited life options; minimal health, nutrition, and education; and the erosion of self-esteem.

The Children's Defense Fund (1985) refers to the problem of adolescent pregnancy in the black community as "a crisis that threatens to cripple economic progress and lock generations of children into poverty." The problem is exacerbated by public income transfer programs that lift women and their children out of poverty at a rate three to five times lower than men (Cassetty & McRoy, 1983). With respect to the association between teenage birthrates and race, Cummings and Cummings (1983) advise that the peculiar mixture of race and sexuality obscures a serious social problem among American youth generally: the lack of assistance from family, schools, and community organizations with respect to decisions concerning sexual and reproductive behavior. These researchers attribute this problem to the disadvantaged and powerless status of minority female populations, which bias the delivery of family-planning services in ways that deprive them of needed assistance.

Infant Death Rates

Infant death rates are commonly used as a measure for assessing the overall health status of a population and prevailing social, economic, and health conditions. In addition to low birth weight, other causes of infant death are congenital anomalies, sudden infant death syndrome, respiratory distress syndrome, and disorders related to short gestation (National Center for Health Statistics, 1984). The survival of an infant through its first month of life (neonatal period) is heavily influenced by biological factors such as the physical condition and nutrition of the mother, and health care factors such as the quality of prenatal care and the delivery environment. Babies born to teenage mothers who have not reached full physical maturity are especially vulnerable in that they are less likely to be fully developed at birth (National Center for Health Statistics, 1984). This problem is exacerbated by the tendency of teenage mothers to avoid or delay seeking prenatal care. The survival of an infant through its first year is heavily dependent on diet, postneonatal medical care, and housing and environmental conditions, such as exposure to vermin and lead poisoning (U.S. Department of Health and Human Services, 1980).

Except for congenital anomalies, the risk of infant death is much higher for black than white infants for all other causes, contributing factors being poverty and the conditions that attend it that place the health of poor women and their children in jeopardy (Weaver, 1976). In addition to environmental and medical factors, such conditions include emotional stress, poor nutrition, health-related habits that reflect a belief in fate and luck, and poor self-concept on the part of many disadvantaged women. Such attitudes mean that many poor mothers tend to minimize the importance of prenatal and postneonatal care, preoccupied as they are with maintenance survival rather than with the prevention of future problems (Rainwater, 1974). Although reflecting the reality of their impoverished existence, such attitudes also serve to compound the problems associated with the provision of timely and accessible health services, problems undoubtedly exacerbated by the lack of health insurance coverage and money. Because disadvantaged women tend to receive inadequate preventive health care and poor prenatal care, and their children less than adequate well-baby care (Weaver, 1976), states' maternal and child health expenditures have been shown to be important in increasing access to pre- and postnatal care and thereby reducing infant death rates, although the present analysis does not speak to maternal and child health expenditures per se.

State Suicide Rates

Various theories have been used to explain suicide phenomena: cultural (Stack, 1979), psychological (Shneidman, 1973; 1980; 1985), economic (Ahlburg & Schapiro, 1983; Brenner, 1984), demographic (Lester & Lester, 1971; Maris, 1969), and social (Durkheim, 1966). Divorce, migration, race, income, unemployment, gender, age, health, and ethnicity have all been found to be associated with suicide. Durkheim developed the construct of social integration to explain societal differences in the incidence of suicide, that is, as being a function of those characteristics of a society's institutions that serve to bind individuals to the larger collectivity. He held that the rate of suicide varies inversely with the degree of social integration in society and that a society having a high incidence of divorce would be considered low on social integration and thus apt to have more people engaging in suicidal behaviors. Other researchers have made the connection between suicide and divorce through psychological states and conditions common in the population of divorced individuals, such as the loss of spousal roles and functions, increased sexual tensions, guilt, emotional hurt, and so forth. Trovato (1986), noting historical differences in the relationship between suicide and divorce, ascribed these differences to the degree of structural change occurring in society at any given time, implying that a high degree of social change accounts for increased rates of family dissolution, and for the individual, severe psychological distress, or in Shneidman's terms, heightened perturbation with the sometimes lethal consequence of suicide.

Occupational status and income level also have been found to be inversely related to suicide (Maris, 1969; Powell, 1958). Income level determines the extent to which human want and needs can be satisfied, low-income levels being related to higher rates of mental illness and depression, and higher levels of dissatisfaction (Hollingshead & Redlich, 1958). Brenner (1984) found a positive association between suicide rates for males ages 15 to 24 and AFDC, suggestive of the frustrated needs of young males living in poor female-headed families. Both the Brenner (1984) and Ahlburg and Schapiro (1983) studies showed that unemployment rates combined with age, particularly with reference to males, are positively related to suicide. Others attribute the increase in suicide associated with age to failing health, the loss of friends and spouse through death, financial difficulties, and the loss of a meaningful life role with retirement (Lester & Lester, 1971). Cultural and socialization theories help to account for the lower incidence of suicide among women and blacks, women being more willing than men to seek help when faced with personal difficulties, and blacks tending to externalize feelings of aggression, as evidenced by higher rates of homicide among blacks, rather than internalizing them as whites tend to do (Hendin, 1969; Seiden, 1970).

METHODS

The Measures

State-level public policy was measured by state per capita expenditures for health, public welfare, and education, and state per capita taxes. State per capita expenditures for health include expenditures for health research, clinics, nursing, immunization, maternal and child health, and other categorical, environmental, and general health services provided by health agencies as well as the establishment and operation of hospital facilities, the provision of hospital care, and the support of other public or private hospitals. Such expenditures do not include vendor payments for health services administered under public welfare programs, or Medicaid or Medicare payments. State per capita expenditures for public welfare include support and assistance to persons in financial and social need, such as cash assistance, vendor payments for medical care, burials, and other commodities and services for persons in financial need, including social services. State per capita expenditures for education include schools, colleges, and other educational institutions and programs for adults, veterans, and other special classes. State per capita expenditures for local schools include direct state payments for the operation of local public schools, construction of school buildings, purchase and operation of school buses, and other local school services. State per capita taxes include all compulsory contributions exacted by state governments for public purposes, such as sales, individual income, corporation net income, property, and death and gift taxes and motor vehicle license fees. It does not include social insurance or employee retirement contributions.

As already indicated, the rewards or costs of public policy were measured by state rates of teenage births, infant mortality, and suicide, lower rates representing favorable outcomes or rewards, and higher rates, unfavorable outcomes or costs. State demographics, as antecedent variables, were measured by the age structure, gender, racial, and household composition of states' populations; marital, employment, and socioeconomic status; and the urbanization and mobility of state populations. Fiscal capacity was measured by states' income level and distribution.

Several measures were used for states' age structure and income distribution. Age measures included median age, the percentage of persons in the 15 to 17 and 18 to 24 age categories, in each ten-year age category thereafter to age 65, and those 65 years of age and over. Income distribution measures included median income, household income, per capita income, the percentage of persons in each income quintile up to $50,000 and over, and the percentage of individuals, families, and children living below the poverty level. Socioeconomic measures included the state percentage of persons with 12 and 16 years of education. Marital status or stability was measured by state divorce rates and employment status by state unemployment rates. Population change and mobility measures included overall rates of population change in terms of people moving in and out of states between 1970 and 1980; the percentage of persons born in the state in which they presently reside; and the percentage of immigrators living in states. Measures of urbanization included the percentage of persons living in urban areas and population density. Racial composition was measured by the percentage of whites, blacks, Asian and South Pacific Islanders, and American Indian, Eskimo, and Aleuts in state populations; and gender composition by the ratio of males to females in states' populations. The percentage of low birth weight babies born to both white and black mothers was included as an additional independent variable for state infant death rates.

Statistical Procedures

All of the data used in the analyses are aggregate state-level data. Data for infant death rates and state suicide rates were gathered for the year 1982. Data for teenage birthrates by state were available only for 1980, not 1982. Data for all of the independent variables were gathered for the year 1980 to allow for the time lag in their effects to show relative to 1982 state infant death and suicide rates. Data sources include the U.S. Bureau of the Census (1983), the Council for State Governments (1982), and the National Center for Health Statistics (1984).

In accordance with the exploratory nature of the study, stepwise regression procedures were used in the analyses of the dependent variables: state rates of teenage births, infant deaths, and suicide. Because population or sample size requirements of multiple regression procedures impose limits on the number of independent variables that can be analyzed in relation to a single dependent variable at any one time, the independent variables were divided into blocks of three or four, the 50 states being the study's population. Although tests of significance are inappropriate when analyzing data based on entire populations, they, together with the strength of bivariate relationships, were used as guides for determining which variables and their measures to include in the multiple regression equations. After analyzing the independent variables in sets to assess their predictive ability relative to the dependent variables, those that emerged as the best predictors within each set were analyzed together to examine their combined effects relative to the variance in the dependent variables, and the contribution of the policy variables to the variance. In the analysis of infant death rates, state health expenditures were entered into the final equation first in order to assess its effects when controlling for the effects of the predictor variables. The same procedure was used in analyzing per capita state expenditures for public welfare in relation to state suicide rates.

Following these analyses, the same statistical procedures were used to examine the relative effects of state fiscal capacity, state demographics, and prevailing attitudes toward public spending on the policy variables. Although the findings from these latter analyses will be discussed, they will not be presented in detail in this paper.

Data used here are limited by the accuracy and reliability of the data-gathering and reporting practices of the individual states and the jurisdictional units that comprise them. This has particular relevance in the case of blacks, particularly black males, who tend to be underreported in census surveys (Cutright, 1986). The data also are limited by their aggregate level of measurement, which means that the findings cannot be generalized to units of analysis other than states. Nor can the findings be used as a basis for drawing conclusions about the effects of specific programs within each of the expenditure categories since such categories include a number of programs. Another limiting feature of the expenditures data is they pertain to state spending defined above, regardless of funding source, state, local, or federal, which means that state effort by itself cannot be identified in this analysis.

The findings describe statistical relationships between and among a set of variables within an exploratory context. No attempt has been made to create or test a hypothesized model of causal relationships, although conceivably the study's findings could become the basis for developing such a model for later testing, and indeed, in this discussion are used as a basis for conjecture about such relationships. Also, despite the stringent controls of multiple regression procedures (Brenner, 1984), the reported relationships could be affected in unobservable ways by variables not included in the analysis. The findings could be biased by human error, despite all good efforts to minimize it. Moreover, the data are subject to the instability inherent in small populations or samples that the 50 states represent. Although age and race variables are included in the analyses, age- and race-specific analyses were not undertaken. This could mask or cloud certain relationships (Cutright, 1986). And since an analysis of state financing of state expenditures was not undertaken, except for state per capita taxes, ambiguities relative to some of the study's findings could also have been created.

RESULTS

Bivariate Relationships: Teenage Birthrates

The bivariate relationships of teenage birthrates are shown in Table 1. While consistent with the findings of other studies, they shed new light on the connections between state teenage birthrates and state-level public policy. In brief, they show that state teenage birthrates are inversely related to state per capita expenditures for both public welfare and education, particularly for local schools, and state per capita taxes. In other words, states that spend less per capita for public welfare and for education, particularly for local schools, and have lower per capita taxes are states that have higher teenage birthrates. The findings also show that states that have higher teenage birthrates are states that spend more per capita on health care. Thus in addition to the costs inherent in higher teenage birthrates, states that spend less for public welfare and education are required to spend more for health care.

Just as other analyses have found teenage birthrates to be strongly and inversely related to educational attainment level (National Center for Health Statistics, 1984), so did the present study; it also found inverse relationships between state teenage birthrates and states' ratio of males to females and median family income. States having higher school dropout rates, lower median family income, and fewer males are states that have higher teen-

Table 1

Zero Order Correlations for State Teenage Birthrates,
Infant Death Rates, and Suicide Rates

	Teenage Birthrate[1]	Infant Deaths[2]	Suicide Rates[2]
Policy Variables			
State per capita expenditures/education	-.34	--	--
State per capita expenditures/public welfare	-.49	--	-.45
State per capita expenditures/health care	.25	.24	--
State per capita expenditures/ for elementary/ secondary schools	-.52	--	-.22
State per capita taxes	-.20	--	--
State per capita expenditures/mental health	--	--	-.22
State per capita expenditures/Title XX	--	--	-.20
Expenditure change/Title XX	--	--	.25
Health Status Variables			
Percent births low birth weight, all races	--	.52	--
Percent births low birth weight, black children	--	.26	--
Family Variables/Marital Status, 1982			
Ratio per 1,000 live births to unmarried women, all races	--	.59	--
Ratio per 1,000 live births to unmarried women, whites	--	-.24	--
Ratio per 1,000 live births to unmarried women, blacks	--	.31	--
Teenage birthrates	--	.36	--
State divorce rates	.23	--	.79
Population Density Variables			
Population per square mile	-.26	--	-.44
Percent state population urban	-.30	--	--
Ethnicity/Race Variables:			
Percent state population white	-.36	-.33	--
Percent state population black	.67	.69	-.25
Percent population American Indian, Eskimo, Aluet	--	--	.27
Gender Variables: Ratio of males to females	-.29	-.28	.40
Mobility Variables: Percent population born in state	.24	--	-.63
State population change rates	--	--	.77
Percent population from other states	--	-.26	.69
Age Variables			
Percent of population 15-17 years	.33	.30	--
Percent of population 65 and over	--	--	-.24
Education Variables			
Percent population 12 years education	-.77	-.48	.28
Percent population 16 years education	-.66	-.26	--
Employment Status Variables			
Percent labor force unemployed	.22	.34	--
Income Variables			
Median family income	-.60	--	--
Percent households with incomes less than $10,000	.68	--	--
Percent households with incomes $10,000 to $19,999	.14	--	.23
Percent households with incomes $20,000 to $29,999	-.59	--	--
Percent households with incomes $30,000 to $39,999	-.51	--	--
Percent households with incomes $40,000 to $49,999	-.43	--	--
Percent households with incomes over $50,000	-.36	--	--
Percent persons whose income is below poverty	.79	.38	--
Percent families whose income is below poverty	.78	.40	--
Percent of female-headed households living in poverty	--	.43	-.24
Percent of children living in poverty	--	.45	--

TABLE 1 (continued)

	Teenage Birthrate[1]	Infant Deaths[2]	Suicide Rates[2]
Community Disorganization Variable: State crime rate	--	--	.32

[1]1980
[2]1982

age birthrates. Also in keeping with the findings of other studies, the present study found positive relationships between state teenage birthrates and state divorce rates, state unemployment rates, the percentage of blacks in state populations (Zelnick & Kantner, 1972), the percentage of families living in poverty, the percentage of persons living in the state in which they were born, and the percentage of 15- to 17-year-olds in state populations. Thus, state demographics, state policy choices, state opportunity and mobility structures (Long, 1975) all were associated with state teenage birthrates in this study. The variables showing the strongest relationship, in order of descending strength, include the percentage of persons and families living in poverty, the percentage of persons with less than 12 years of education, the percentage of blacks, and states' per capita expenditures for local schools and public welfare (see Table 1).

Predictors of State Teenage Birthrates

The variables that emerged as predictors of state teenage birthrates were the policy and opportunity variables: state per capita expenditures for public welfare, the percentage of families living below poverty, the percentage of state populations that had completed 12 years of education, and state unemployment rates. These four variables together accounted for .81 of the explained variance in state teenage birthrates, with state per capita expenditures for public welfare showing a relatively strong influence, beta = $-.35$ (S.E. = .08; see Table 2). The negative direction of the relationship indicates that *low* rather than high expenditures for public welfare combined with a high percentage of families living in poverty, a higher percentage of persons not completing 12 years of education, and high state unemployment rates are all associated with high state teenage birthrates. These findings are consistent with those of other studies (Chilman, 1980; Ross & Sawhill, 1975) and, like them, tend to refute the commonly held view that public welfare benefits encourage teenagers to have babies for the purpose of acquiring welfare status.

Conversely, high state expenditures for public welfare combined with a low percentage of families living in poverty, a high percentage of persons completing 12 years of education, and low state unemployment rates are predictive of *low* teenage birthrates. This means that state per capita spending for public welfare, which includes not only states' share of financial participation in AFDC, but also the funding of many related services, could be a function of the number of persons whose needs must be met within the fiscal capacities of states and their legislated allocations. This is a distinct possibility in light of the inverse relationship between state per capita expenditures for public welfare and the percentage of families living in poverty, $r = -.26$ (see Table 3). However, an analysis of the predictors of such expenditures suggests that this is *not* the case, using any of the income measures incorporated in the study as proxies for state fiscal capacity. Although positively associated with state spending for public welfare, the income level of state populations was not a predictor of it. Thus, while high teenage birthrates indeed

Table 2

Standardized Regression Coefficients of Predictors of Outcomes

	Beta	Standard Error/Beta	Adjusted R^2
Teenage Birth Rates (1980)			
Percent families below poverty	.37	.10	.60
State per capita expenditures, public welfare	-.35	.06	.69
Education, 12 years	-.39	.10	.77
State unemployment rates	.17	.07	.80
Infant Death Rates (1982)			
State per capita expenditures, health	-.09	.11	.04
Percentage of population, black	.69	.11	.46
Percent labor force unemployed	.21	.10	.50
Suicide Rates (1982)			
State per capita expenditures, public welfare	.07	.10	.19
State divorce rates	.53	.12	.63
State population change rates	.38	.13	.67
Percent population, income $10,000 to $19,999	.23	.09	.71

may contribute to state poverty rates, as many assert, low per capita expenditures for public welfare do too, as many others also assert and have observed in other contexts as well (Duncan, 1984; IRP Focus, 1985; Zimmerman, 1985).

That a higher percentage of families living in poverty is inversely related to state public welfare expenditures and to state school completion rates and all are predictors of state teenage birthrates highlights the interrelatedness of these phenomena. As can be seen in Table 2, all three are almost equally strong in their ability to predict state teenage birthrates. These findings together with those showing positive relationships between state teenage birthrates, state unemployment rates, and the percentage of fam-

Table 3

Correlation Matrices: Variables in Regressions

Teenage Birth Rates, 1980

	Teen birthrates	Families/ poverty	Public welfare expenditures	Education 12 years	Unemployment rates
Teen birthrates	1.00	.78	-.49	-.77	.22
Families/Poverty	.78	1.00	-.26	-.74	.18
Public welfare expenditures	-.49	-.26	1.00	.17	.27
Education, 12 years	-.77	-.74	.17	1.00	-.33
Unemployment Rates	.22	.18	.27	-.21	1.00

Infant Death Rates, 1982

	Infant deaths	Health expenditures	Percent black	Percent unemployed
Infant deaths	1.00	.24	.69	.34
Per capita health expenditures, 1980	.24	1.00	.46	.07
Percent population black	.69	.46	1.00	.19
Percent unemployed	.34	.07	.19	1.00

State Suicide Rates, 1982

	Suicide rates	Welfare expenditures	Population change rates	Divorce rates	Income $10-19,999
Suicide rates	1.00	-.45	.76	.79	.23
Per capita welfare expenditures	-.45	1.00	-.53	-.42	-.41
Population change	.76	-.53	1.00	.76	.07
Divorce rates	.79	-.42	.76	1.00	.00
Percent income $10,000-$19,999	.23	-.41	.07	.00	1.00

ilies living in poverty depict state opportunity structures so deficient in the options they offer poor teenagers that in such states, poor teenagers indeed may perceive early childbearing and accelerated parenthood as the only viable ones for obtaining the outcome or reward they are seeking: adult status. Low expenditures for public welfare can hardly help matters. That states' school completion rates are predictive of states' teenage birthrates and the former are inversely related to states' expenditures for education suggests that while such expenditures may not be predictive of states' teenage birthrates, they could affect them indirectly.

Bivariate Relationships: Infant Death Rates

The bivariate relationships for infant death rates are shown in Table 1. Consistent with data from other studies, they show that state infant death rates are positively related to state teenage birthrates and low birth weight babies, the latter two variables being very strongly and positively related to each other. State infant death rates also are positively related to per capita state expenditures for health care, but not to any of the other policy variables. Because states are required to provide health care to medically indigent persons and state infant death rates are strongly associated with state poverty rates, expenditures for health care necessarily would be greater in states having higher infant death rates. However, the relationship though positive is not as strong as might be expected, $r = .24$. Other findings indicate that just as states that have fewer males have higher teenage birthrates, such states also have higher infant death rates. Higher infant death rates also are inversely related to population change and mobility as measured by the percentage of persons in-migrating to states in which they presently reside which means that states having fewer people in-migrating to them are states that have higher infant death rates. Thus, the absence of social and economic mobility is associated with both state infant death rates and teenage birthrates.

Both of the educational attainment variables are related to state infant death rates, as they are to state teenage birth rates, and in the same negative direction, although not as strongly in the case of the former as in the latter. Contrary to state teenage birthrates, which were related to almost all of the income measures, state infant death rates are related only to the poverty measures. Not only is the relationship between state infant death rates limited to the poverty measures, as opposed to other income measures, its relationship is not as strong as the relationship of teenage birthrates to these measures. While the ratio of births for unmarried women relative to married women for all races shows a strong relationship to states' infant death rates, the relationship is positive for blacks but negative for whites. Consistent with these findings and those of other studies, the positive relationship between state infant death rates and the percentage of blacks in states' populations underscores the importance of race in state infant death rates.

Given the strong positive relationship between state teenage birthrates and infant death rates, it is hardly surprising that both are similarly related to many of the same variables: high poverty rates, low school-completion rates, high unemployment rates, low population mobility rates, and high state per capita expenditures for health care.

Predictors of State Infant Death Rates

Consistent with data from other studies, the strongest predictor of state infant death rates by far was the percentage of blacks in state populations followed by state unemployment rates, as shown in Table 2. Together these two variables accounted for 52 percent of the total explained variance in infant death rates. Although state per capita expenditures for health care positively are related to state infant death rates, their effects were practically nonexistent when controlling for the other two variables. This does not mean that such expenditures are unimportant relative to infant death rates, but rather that their importance is not revealed in this analysis, perhaps because of the comprehensive nature of the expenditure measure itself, or by variables not taken into account in the analysis. The analysis, after all, leaves 48 percent of the variance in state infant death rates unexplained. On the other hand, it also may be the case that states' health expenditures relative to infant death rates in fact were insufficient to overcome the strong effects of race and unemployment rates in 1980. This possibility is very real when consideration is given to the way in which health care is financed in this country, largely through third party insurance payments, federal block grants to states, and special purpose federal grants, such as maternal and child health grants. Indeed in 1985, states paid the smallest share of the country's total health care costs, the largest share being paid by private insurance carriers, the next largest by the federal government, and the third largest by individuals and families themselves (American Public Welfare Association, 1986). For poor women without health insurance, such financing presents serious problems with respect to obtaining health care for themselves and their children.

The correlation matrix in Table 3 shows the interrelationship among the variables in the regression equation with infant death rates. The weak relationship between state infant death rates and state unemployment rates and between state unemployment rates and the percentage of blacks in state populations could well reflect the underreporting of black males in state populations. It also could reflect the way unemployment is officially defined in that only active job seekers are defined and counted as unemployed. This means that inactive job seekers who, in discouragement, have given up looking for a job they cannot find, are not included in the count.

Bivariate Relationships: State Suicide Rates

Most of the findings of the present research are consistent with those of other studies. State suicide rates are strongly related to each of the mobility measures included in the study, positively related to both state population change rates and the percentage of state populations that inmigrated to the state in which they live, and inversely related to the percentage of state populations that live in the state which they were born, as shown in Table 1. State suicide rates also are strongly and positively related to state divorce rates, and positively but less strongly related to the ratio of males to females, to ethnicity, that is the percentage of American Indian, Eskimo and Aleut in state populations, and to state crime rates, all consistent with Durkheim's social integration theory.

As Table 1 shows, state suicide rates also are positively related to the percentage of state populations having annual incomes between $10,000 and $19,999, and the percentage of state populations having attained 12 years of education, relationships dissimilar from those pertaining to state teenage birthrates and infant death rates. Like state teenage birthrates, however, state suicide rates are inversely related to per capita state expenditures for public welfare, but much more strongly. They also are inversely related to the percentage of blacks in state populations and the percentage of female-headed households, consistent with findings from other studies, and inversely related to population density and the percentage of persons 65 years and older, consistent with Preston's recent analysis (1984).

Thus, it appears that while state suicide rates are related to many of the same variables as state teenage birthrates and infant death rates, the pattern of these relationships is different in the case of state suicide rates. For example, while state rates of high school completion are *inversely* related to teenage birthrates and infant death rates, they are *positively* related to state suicide rates. That high school completion rates are positively associated with state suicide rates, however, speaks not to the adverse effects of education, but rather to the frustrated needs of moderately educated individuals in high suicide rate states. A Durkheimian perspective suggests that this has to do with structures and mechanisms for social integration that apparently are absent or weakened in states that have highly mobile populations and large populations without strong family ties. That state rates of college completion are *not* associated with state suicide rates points to the value of higher educational attainment levels for coping with problems on both individual and state levels, an interpretation supported by the positive relationship between state rates of college completion and state spending for mental health services.

The mobility measures reveal a pattern of relationships similar to that of state rates of high school completion with respect to state teenage birthrates, infant death rates, and suicide rates. Inversely related to state infant death rates and state teenage birthrates, the mobility measures are positively related to state suicide rates. This means that states having a higher percentage of persons who live in the state in which they were born have higher teenage birthrates and infant death rates while states having a larger percentage of persons who moved into the state in which they reside have higher suicide rates. Also, state divorce rates play a much stronger role in state suicide rates than they do in state teenage birthrates, poverty playing a stronger role in the latter.

Predictors of State Suicide Rates

The predictors of state suicide rates are shown in Table 2. Per capita state expenditures for public welfare, although showing a relatively strong inverse bivariate relationship to state suicide rates, did not prove to be a predictor when controlling for the effects of state divorce rates, state population change rates, and the percentage of persons with annual incomes between $10,000 and $19,999. The latter three variables account for .73 of the explained variance in state suicide rates, state divorce rates being the strongest predictor, beta = .53, followed by state population change rates. Thus, despite its strong inverse bivariate relationship to state suicide rates, it might appear that per capita state expenditures for public welfare are of little or no consequence insofar as state suicide rates are concerned, when taking into account the effects of such powerful predictor variables. Subsequent analysis, however, shows that state per capita expenditures for public welfare are indirectly related to state suicide rates, the combined indirect effects of per capita public welfare expenditures and population change rates, divorce rates, and low income relative to state suicide rates being − .49. These effects suggest that such expenditures indeed are of considerable importance insofar as state suicide rates are concerned and probably of greater importance than commonly realized. That such expenditures represent the kinds of services needed in high suicide rate states is not only supported by the suicide rates themselves, but by the positive relationship between state spending for public welfare and mental health services.

The correlation matrix showing the interrelationships among the predictors of state suicide rates reveals how strongly state divorce rates, state population change rates, and state suicide rates are related to each other (see Table 3). The anomaly in this configuration is the population with incomes between $10,000 and $19,999, which while related to state suicide rates is not related to either state population change rates or state divorce rates. In another context, this group might be described as the working poor. This population is of particular interest because it is singular as an income group in its relationship to state suicide rates. Moreover, states having a larger percentage of persons in this income group have a higher percentage of persons who voted for the leading party in the 1980 presidential election, spend less for public welfare, education, and health care, and levy lower per capita taxes.

Per Capita Spending for Education

Given that state-level public policy seems to promote individual and family well-being when state expenditures for public welfare and education are higher but not when they are lower, what are the important variables that influence such spending choices? To answer a question with a question beginning with state per capita expenditures for education, why do low-spending education states not spend more for education, given that such spending is so highly and positively related to school completion rates and school completion rates are so positively related to income, both of which are so strongly negatively related to both state teenager birthrates and infant death rates? Perhaps the answer to these questions lies in the predictors of such spending: state per capita taxes, state spending for highways, and the ratio of males to females. These three variables together accounted for 90 percent of the total explained variance in state spending for education. All three variables not only are positively related to such spending, but also to each other. In other words, states that spend more for education have a higher ratio of males in their populations, spend more for highways, a mobility variable, and levy higher per capita taxes than states that spend less for education. Low-spending education states, on the other hand, have a higher ratio of females, spend less for highways, and levy lower per capita taxes. Thus, although positively related to such spending and contrary to what might have been expected using any of the income measures incorporated in the study as noted earlier, state fiscal capacity was *not* a predictor of it, nor were prevailing attitudes towards public spending.

Because gender *was* a predictor of such spending, and indeed, related to all of the policy variables, perhaps gender is what accounts for these spending choices. Indeed, in states in which there is a higher ratio of males, both state per capita spending for education and state income level are higher. That these variables are interrelated suggests that states that invest more in education enjoy higher income levels, in part it would seem because they invest more in education, have more males, and males have higher earning capacities than females. (In 1980, males outnumbered females in five states: Wyoming, Nevada, North Dakota, Hawaii, and Alaska. In the remaining 45 states, the ratio of males to 100 females ranged from a low of 90.5 in New York to a high of 99.7 in Idaho.) The effects of gender relative to spending for education also could be a function of age as well as income since women tend to live longer than men. Older age together with lower-income levels could help to account for lower spending for education in states that have a higher ratio of females to males. Thus, to the extent that gender may bias state spending for education, at least two possibilities come to mind. One is that if low-spending education states made a larger investment in education, they too might enjoy the higher income levels of higher spending education states, despite having more females in their populations, assuming that they modified their occupational and wage structures in ways that no longer disadvantage women. At the same time, given that a higher ratio of females to males in state populations is predictive of lower per capita state expenditures for education, and that this relationship could be a function of both age and income, state demographics it would seem place children living in such states at a serious disadvantage relative to children in other states, a phenomenon to which Martha Ozawa (1986) recently called attention. Indeed, their very futures could be at stake, as the positive relationship between state per capita spending for education and school completion rates suggests, given the latter's inverse predictive relationship to state teenage birthrates. In that state spending for education and highways is positively related to the ratio of males to females, and negatively related to the percentage of blacks in state populations, the same speculations apply to the effects of race relative to state spending for education, r = − .27, as apply to gender.

Per Capita State Spending for Public Welfare

The same kinds of questions may be asked about state expenditures for public welfare as were asked about spending for education. Given its inverse relationship to state teenage birthrates and the interrelationships between these rates, state poverty rates, and high school completion rates, why do low-spending welfare states not spend more for the life-maintaining purposes to which such spending is directed? While large populations of poor families may represent a fiscal drain on state finances and hence account for lower per capita state effort, the data from this study, as noted earlier, suggest otherwise. Further, although they were positively related to such spending, it will be recalled that none of the income measures incorporated in the study of state fiscal capacity were predictors of state welfare spending, just as they were not predictors of spending for education. The variables that were predictors of state per capita public welfare spending were: per capita state spending for local schools, the percentage of female-headed households, and the percentage of persons voting for the leading party in the 1980 presidential election, as a measure of prevailing attitudes toward public spending. These three variables together accounted for 61 percent of the total explained variance in state per capita spending for public welfare, state per capita expenditures for local schools being the strongest predictor and positively related to it.

The percentage of female-headed households, which was the third predictor of public welfare expenditures, was weakly related to only a few of the income measures in the study; positively in the case of states' median income and annual income between $30,000 and $40,000, and negatively in the case of annual income between $10,000 and $20,000, indicating again that fiscal considerations do not predominate in choices concerning public welfare expenditures. However, because these data are not entirely consistent with data showing the prevalence of poverty among female-headed households, caution should be taken in drawing conclusions about the gender/income relationship from these latter findings. Since the data on female-headed households include all households headed by women, which may include households with multiple earners and older women, other factors may come into play to distort these relationships.

Per Capita State Taxes

With respect to decisions about taxes to support expenditure choices, although the relationships were not as strong as might be supposed, states that levy higher per capita taxes are states that spend more for education, public welfare, and highways. Thus it is true that such choices represent costs for individual taxpayers, short-run costs that yield long-term gains, given the implications of the positive relationships between state spending for education and public welfare and states' high school completion rates, for states' teenage birthrates and infant death rates, and for states' fiscal capacity as measured by the percentage of persons with higher incomes. However, in assessing the importance of state fiscal capacity relative to states' tax choices, the data again show that state fiscal capacity was *not* a predictor of such choices. The primary and really only predictor of state per capita taxes was state expenditures for education. It alone accounted for .73 of the total explained variance in state per capita taxes, state expenditures for public welfare contributing an additional .10 when controlling for the effects of expenditures for education, an influence that would not have been noticed had that of spending for education not been controlled. Thus it would appear that states that spend more for education do so without undue regard for fiscal capacity, that they generate the revenues they need to finance their choices and not the other way around. Contrary to expectations, prevailing attitudes toward public spending were *not* related to state per capita taxes.

SUMMARY AND CONCLUSION

State expenditures for education and public welfare seem to promote individual and family well-being in states that spend more in these areas, but in states that spend less they seem to reflect the same social malaise that state teenage birthrates, infant death rates, and state suicide rates themselves represent. The findings highlight the central importance of education and adequate income and security for individual and family well-being — and for states' as well — and also point to the critical role that state-level public policy can play in this regard. The findings indicate that if low-spending public welfare and education states were to spend more, they may be able to raise their school completion rates and lower their poverty rates, teenage birthrates, and infant death rates.

The findings also highlight the conflicting influences that enter into states' spending choices. Although they suggest that spending choices are informed by a general awareness of their implications for individual and family well-being, and do take into account information about changing family structures and needs (or that there is more support for such spending in states that do), they are also influenced by prevailing attitudes toward lower public spending. Such attitudes are important predictors of collective choice with respect to such state budget items as public welfare.

The findings raise interesting and important questions with respect to state suicide rates. What is the meaning of the inverse relationship of *all* of the predictors of state suicide rates, and state suicide rates themselves, to state spending for public welfare, and the positive relationship of *all* of these variables to negative attitudes toward public spending, assuming that the indicator used in this analysis is a valid measure of such attitudes? Do these relationships mean that the norm of reciprocity is *not* the norm in states that are characterized by high rates of suicide, high rates of mobility, and high rates of divorce? The data from this study certainly would support such a conclusion. These relationships are not perfect, however, in that states with more stable populations spend less for public welfare too — and have higher rates of teenage births and infant deaths. Public welfare expenditures aside, is there something inherent in mobility phenomena that fosters higher state suicide rates on the one hand and higher state teenage birthrates on the other, with gender and race as central components? What is the thread that connects these phenomena, particularly in light of their inverse relationship to states' spending choices?

Although the findings of this study on the relationship between state-level public policy and individual and family well-being raise as many questions as they answer, they are consistent with choice and exchange theories in that states' avoidance of costs in the form of low expenditures for public welfare is shown to be costly in terms of teenage birthrates and higher levels of social malaise. Low spending for education by states compounds the problem, creating barriers to the opportunities that minorities and women need for upward mobility. Such choices on the part of low-spending states also erode the quality of life for all of the individuals and families that constitute their populations. Further, they violate the norm of reciprocity, hurting rather than helping those who need the opportunities such expenditures would aid. Whether other choices are possible in states in which the norm of reciprocity may be dormant or undeveloped is highly questionable. It is for this reason that the diminished role of the federal government in human affairs should be viewed with alarm, connoting as it does a violation of the norm at the highest of governmental levels.

REFERENCES

Ahlburg, D. & Schapiro, M. (1983). *Socio-economic ramifications of changing cohort size: An analysis and forecast of U.S. post-war suicide rates by age and sex*. Minneapolis, MN: Industrial Relations Center, University of Minnesota.

Baldwin, W. (1984). *Adolescent pregnancy and childbearing: rates, trends and research findings*. The Center for Population Research, NICHD, May.

Book of the States (1982). Lexington, KY: Council on State Governments.

Brenner, H. (1984). *Estimating the effects of economic change on national health and social well-being*. A study prepared for the use of the subcommittee on economic goals and intergovernmental policy of the Joint Economic Congress of the United States, June 15. Washington, DC: U.S. Government Printing Office.

Cassetty, J. & McRoy, R. (1983). Gender, race, and the shrinking welfare dollar. *Public Welfare, 41* Summer: 36-39.

Chilman, C. S. (1980). Social and psychological research concerning adolescent childbearing: 1970-1980. *Journal of Marriage and Family, 42*: 793-805.

Chilman, C. S. (1983). *Adolescent sexuality in a changing American society: Social and psychological perspectives*. New York: John Wiley & Sons, Inc.

Cohen, M. W. & Freidman, S. B. (1975). Nonsexual motivation of adolescent sexual behavior. *Medical Aspects of Human Sexuality, 9*: 8-31.

Cummings M. & Cummings, S. (1983). Family planning among the urban poor: Sexual politics and social policy. *Family Relations, 32*: 47-58.

Cutright, P. (1972). The teenage sexual revolution and the myth of an abstinent past. *Family Planning Perspectives*, 3: 26-47.

Cutright, P. (1986). Personal correspondence. August 21.

Cvetkovich, G. & Grote, B. (1979). Psychological maturity, ego identity and fertility-related behavior. Paper presented at the American Psychological Meeting. New York: September.

Cvetkovich, B. & Grote, B. (1980). Psychosocial development and the social problem of teenage illegitimacy. In C. S. Chilman (Ed.), *Adolescent pregnancy and childbearing*, Washington, DC: U. S. Government Printing Office.

Dembo, M. H. & Lundell, B. (1979). Factors affecting adolescent contraception practices: Implications for sex education. *Adolescence*, 14: 657-664.

Durkheim, E. (1966). *Suicide*. New York: Free Press.

Duncan, G. (1984). *Years of poverty/Years of plenty*. Ann Arbor, MI: University of Michigan, Institute for Social Research.

Dye, T. (1966). *Politics, economics, and the public*. Chicago, IL: Rand McNally and Company.

Ekeh, P. (1974). *Social exchange theory*. Cambridge, MA: Harvard University Press.

Erikson, E. (1968). *Identity, youth and crisis*. New York: W. W. Norton and Company.

Eulau, H. & Eyestone R. (1968). Policy maps of city councils and policy outcomes: A developmental analysis. *American Political Science Review*, 62: 124-143.

Gottschalk, L. A., Titchener, J. L., Piker, H. N. & Stewart, S. S. (1964). Psychosocial factors associated with pregnancy in adolescent girls: A preliminary report. *Journal of Nervous and Mental Diseases*, 138: 524-534.

Gouldner, A. (1960). The norm of reciprocity. *American Sociological Review*, 25: 161-178.

Hendin, H. (1969). *Black suicide*. New York: Basic Books.

Hollingshead, A. B. & Redlich, F. (1958). *Social class and mental illness*. New York: Wiley and Sons.

IRP Focus (1984). Madison, WI: Institute for Research on Poverty, 1: 5.

Knapp, E. S. (1982). Trends in state legislation: 1980-81. In *Book of the states: 1982-83*. Lexington, KY: Council of State Governments.

Kreipe, R. E. (1983). Prevention of adolescent pregnancy: A developmental approach. In E. R. McAnarney (Ed.), *Premature adolescent pregnancy and parenthood*. New York: Grune and Stratton.

Lester, D. & Lester, G. (1971). *Suicide: The gamble with death*. Englewood Cliffs, NJ: Prentice-Hall.

Levi-Straus, C. (1969). *The elementary structures of kinship*. Boston, MA: Beacon Press.

Long, L. H. (1975). Poverty status and receipt of welfare among migrants and nonmigrants in large cities. In K. Kammeyer (Ed.), *Population studies*. Chicago, IL: Rand McNally College Publishing Co.

Maris, R. W. (1969). *Social forces in urban suicide*. Homewood, IL: Dorsey Press.

Moore, K. A. & Burt, M. (1982). *Private crisis, public costs: Policy perspectives on teenage childbearing*. Washington, DC: The Urban Institute.

National Center for Health Statistics (1984a). Advance report, final mortality statistics, 1982. *Monthly Vital Statistics Report*. Vol. 33, No. 9, Supp. DHHS Pub. No. (DHS) 85-1120. Hyattsville, MD: Public Health Service, December 20.

National Center for Health Statistics, S. J. Ventura (1984). Trends in teenage childbearing, United States, 1970-81. *Vital and Health Statistics* Series 21, No. 41. DHS Pub. No. (PHS) 84-1919. Public Health Services. Washington, DC: U.S. Government Printing Office, September.

Nye I. (1979). Choice, exchange and the family. In W. Burr, R. Hill, I. Nye, & I. Reiss (Eds.), *Contemporary theories about the family*, Vol. 2. New York: Free Press.

Olson, M. (1974). *The logic of collective action*. Cambridge, MA: Harvard University Press.

Ozawa, M. (1986). Nonwhites and the demographic imperative in social welfare spending. *Social Work. 31* 6: 440-447.

Piaget, J. (1967). *Six psychological studies*. New York: Vintage.

Powell, E. (1958). Occupation, status, and suicide: Towards a redefinition of anomie. *American Sociological Review, 23*: 131-139.

Preston, S. (1984). Children and the elderly: Divergent paths for America's dependent. *Demography 21*: 435-457.

Preventing Children Having Children (1985). Washington, DC: Children's Defense Fund.

Rainwater, L. (1974). The lower class: health, illness, and medical institutions. In L. Rainwater (Ed.), *Inequality and justice*. Chicago, IL: Aldine Publishing Co.

Ross. H. & Sawhill, I. (1975). *Time of transition: The growth of families headed by women*. Washington, DC: The Urban Institute.

Shneidman, E. S. (1973). Suicide. In *Encyclopedia Britannica*. Chicago, IL: William Genton: 383-385.

Shneidman, E. S. (1980). *Voices of death*. New York: Harper and Row.

Shneidman, E. S. (1985). *Definition of suicide*. New York: John Wiley and Sons.

Stack, Steven (1979). Immigration of suicide. Paper presented at 12th annual meeting of the American Association of Suicidology. Denver, Colorado.

Terrell, P. (1986). Taxing the poor. *Social Service Review, 60*: 272-286.

This Week in Washington (1986). The American Public Welfare Association, August 1.

Trovato, F. (1986). The relationship between marital dissolution and suicide: The Canadian case. *Journal of Marriage and Family. 48*: 341-348.

U. S. Bureau of the Census (1983). *County and city data book*. Washington, DC: U. S. Government Printing Office.

U. S. Department of Health and Human Services (HHS) (1980). *Health: United States, 1980*. PHS 81-1232, December.

Weaver, J. V. (1976). *National health policy and the underserved: Ethnic minorities, women, and the elderly*. St. Louis, MO: The C. V. Mosby Co.

Wiiensky, H. (1975). *The welfare state and inequality*. Los Angeles, CA: University of California Press.

Zelnik, M. & Kantner, J. F. (1972). Sexual and contraceptive experiences of young unmarried women in the United States, 1976 and 1971. *Family Planning Perspectives. 4*: 9-18.

Zimmerman, S. L. (1985). Families and economic policies: An instrumental perspective. *Social Casework. 66*: 424-431.

Is Being Poor
a Mental Health Hazard?

Freda L. Paltiel, MPH

SUMMARY. From a perspective of needs, risks and tasks of women throughout the life and family cycle the paper examines relationships between mental health and poverty by reviewing observed determinants and concomitants of poverty as well as stressors and risks associated with women's socioeconomic position, environmental conditions, and social roles. As a tool for policy development, a three-anchor needs proposition and a coping schema and formula are proposed as a new conceptual framework for appraising women's hazards and strengths. The poverty status of women in Canada is also reviewed.

Female poverty can begin with or result from being a failure-to-thrive infant in a family where male babies are preferred (WHO/UNICEF, 1986); a culturally deprived childhood (Boodoosingh & Brown, 1986); an adolescence in a low-socio-economic status (SES) family, especially if, despite high mental ability, the educational expectations for university are low compared with males of the same class or females of medium and high SES families (Porter et al., 1973); a low-paying or an unstable dead-end job in the secondary labor market, unemployment or underemployment; plant or mine closures; foreclosures; technological change; economic dependency on a man who can't or won't share his income or assets; immature motherhood, widowhood or separation, divorce with children and poor enforcement of maintenance obligations (Weitzman, 1985); chronic disease or

Freda L. Paltiel is Senior Adviser, Status of Women, Health and Welfare Canada, Room 2100, Jeanne Mance Building, Ottawa, Ontario, Canada K1A OK9.

The views expressed are those of the author and do not necessarily represent those of the Government of Canada or Health and Welfare Canada.

disability; chemical dependency; natural disasters (Bolin, 1982); migration; an old-age based on past earning and income deficits with inadequate income security entitlements (Paltiel, 1982); systemic discrimination, or any combination of these.

This paper is data-based but not data-bound. Women's salient experience has not been sufficiently studied in a systematic way to provide the answers. We seek evidence for our gut feelings and commonsense knowledge. Psychosocial aspects of health are still an underdeveloped area of research and practice; moreover *mental health* (Leighton, 1982), *poverty* (Stats Can, 1986) and even *mental illness* (Sarwer-Foner, 1983) still lack precise definition. One fact, however, is irrefutable: women are overrepresented among the poor, however identified. Indeed the mountain of documentation produced by the end of the International Women's decade yielded one principal finding: throughout the world, women are overworked and undervalued and, as we are beginning to see, the relationship between women's work and women's worth has profound consequences for their mental health.

The classic Hollingshead and Redlich study (1958) established that significant associations exist between class position and mental illness for both sexes and for all adult age groups, as well as for males but not for females under 15 years of age. Stressors for female adolescents of all social classes deserve greater study (Stavrakaki, 1985).

Buck summarizes the obstacles, deficits and threats to health inherent in poverty: it is the poor who are exposed to dangerous environments, who, if employed, often have stressful, unrewarding and depersonalizing work, who lack the necessities and amenities of life and, who, because they are not part of the mainstream of society, are isolated from information and support. She concludes that above all, poverty is intrinsically debasing and alienating (Buck, 1986). Moreover lower-class persons by virtue of their life circumstances are exposed to more stressors, and with fewer resources to manage them and greater vulnerability to stressors, are doubly victimized (Liem & Liem, 1981).

Money is not a guarantor of mental health, nor does its absence necessarily lead to mental illness. However, it is generally conceded that poverty can be both a determinant and a consequence of poor mental health (Langner & Michael, 1963). The latter is most clearly evidenced in the deinstitutionalized long-term mentally disabled, returned to so-called "communities" without sufficient or appropriate community supports or services. The most tragic of these societal "pushouts" are the homeless "bag ladies."

In the Midtown Manhattan Study (Langner & Michael, 1963) economic deprivation was an important determinant of poorer mental health of low SES persons. Moreover, Hollingshead (1975) found his revisited poorest people (Class V) to be so far removed from community opinion, so much preoccupied with their own affairs that discrimination against their children was personalized against the teacher or school, resulting in premature school withdrawal.

Recently, Canada's Minister of National Health and Welfare noted that:

> Perhaps as a society we deliberately "forget" mental health, because of a certain stigma which remains attached to the subject. The links between the physical, emotional, mental and spiritual planes of human life are profound and intricate. I suspect that we need more research into these linkages, and beyond them into the whole effect of our socio-economic environment on mental health. (Epp, 1986, p. 7)

Indeed, the concept of "Women, Health and Development" (WHD) has become an expression to denote the complex interrelationships between the health of women and their social, political, cultural and economic situations. Studies tell us that women report greater emotional distress than men, and are more often hospitalized for mental health problems, are less likely to take their own lives, but more likely to attempt to do so (and are probably held back by concern for survivors). What follows is an examination of the relationship between mental health and poverty from a perspective of needs, risks and tasks of women throughout the life and family cycles.

Elsewhere, I have written:

> While definitive concepts of mental health are elusive, Freud's simple criteria of the ability to love and to work form a basis. (Eidelberg has adapted Freud's dictum to in-

clude the notion of reciprocity: i.e. to love, to be loved). In search for mental health norms, the risks of subjective judgments and psychiatric labelling reflecting cultural bias, class bias and sex-role bias become apparent if we examine the recurrent criteria of (1) freedom from psychiatric symptoms, (2) a sense of contentment, (3) effective performance in major social roles. (Paltiel, 1977, p. v)

Social roles are not randomly distributed nor necessarily freely undertaken. Penfold and Walker (1983) have shown how psychiatry reinforces women's traditional roles. Dr. Halfdan Mahler, Director-General of the World Health Organization (WHO), in addressing the U.N. Women's Decade World Conference in Nairobi, stated that: "Experts speak indeed of the feminization of poverty, and even in countries where — by legislation, constitution and ideology — women are proclaimed equal, one does not see them where the power is."

SOCIOECONOMIC STATUS OF WOMEN: THE CANADIAN EXPERIENCE

When we look at the distribution of Canadian women across the socioeconomic spectrum, we note first their overrepresentation among the low-income population. In 1985, though 51% of the population, they were 57% of all low-income people. Indeed the incidence of low income in Canada has become feminized, with families headed by women and women who live alone (particularly elderly women) making up a disproportionately large share.

Statistics Canada Low-Income thresholds,* while not official poverty lines, identify the groups that are relatively worse off. In 1985, Low-Income Cut-offs for a two-person family in an urban area (500,000 +) was $13,500, and over $18,000 (all figures are in Canadian dollars) for a three-member family. While 13% of

---

*Defined as those who spend at least 58.5% of their income on food, shelter and clothing. These limits vary by population of area of residence (i.e., urban vs. rural) and by size of the family. They are not intended as measures of "poverty" (Statistics Canada, 1986).

all families were in the low-income category in 1985, representing a drop from 14.5% in 1984, just over 60% of all female lone parents with minors were low income and this proportion has risen steadily since 1981. They constitute 4.5% of all families, but 13.7% of all low-income families in 1985.

The median annual income of all female lone parents in 1984 was just below $15,000, compared to nearly $38,000 for all husband-wife families. Younger women, 24 years old or less, who head families are at very high risk for low-income status, with a median annual income of just $8,747.

In 1985, children under 16 made up 29% or 1.1 million of the low-income population. About one in five (19.2%) Canadian children under 16 years of age were members of low-income families, an increase in 1981, but a decrease from 1984. Although the incidence of low income among single individuals of all ages (37%) has gone down since 1983, this rate is higher for women (42%) than for men (30%). Moreover, unattached women are much more likely to have low incomes in their old age (50%), despite social security measures which have been successful in reducing the rate of low income among elderly unattached individuals. Nearly three out of ten low-income individuals (29%) in 1985 were elderly women, a total of 289,000 women. Since 1980 the rate of low income for all unattached elderly (80% of whom are women) has dropped steadily from 62% to 46%.

In 1984, out of the 5.2 million women in the Canadian labor force, nearly four million were concentrated in the service (46%), trade (18%) and manufacturing (12%) sectors. In the 1983 Annual Review, the Economic Council of Canada found there is still a very substantial clustering of women in the lowest-paid occupations and that the average earnings of the women in these occupations in 1981 was just 64% of the earnings of men in the same jobs ($6,076 vs. $9,559). Moreover, women accounted for 71% of the growing part-time employed labor force in 1984 and over a quarter of all employed women worked part-time, compared with only 7.7% of their male counterparts.

The labor force participation rates of women and men are positively related to educational attainment. However, regardless of education, women's income levels are consistently substantially lower than those of men with the same education. The Women's Bureau of Labour Canada (1986) reported that in 1983 women with a university degree still received an average income ($20,107) that was only slightly higher than that of men with some high school ($19,244) but was actually less than that of male high school graduates ($24,321). So while Canada has legislation in three jurisdictions governing equal pay for work of equal value, pay rates in Canada, as elsewhere, are still largely determined by the sex of the worker, rather than the value of the work. Evidently women's worth is less than men's.

According to Statistics Canada, 1985, average unemployment rates for women living in families with no husband present (14.5%) or whose husbands were not working during the year (17.2%) were much higher than the average for all women in families (11.2%). When dependent children (under 16) were added to the picture, these high rates of unemployment worsened significantly — to over 18% for women with no husband present and 21% for those with nonemployed husbands.

With few exceptions, studies of unemployment have dealt with the male experience. The Canadian Mental Health Association's (CMHA) report on the human costs of unemployment (Kirsh, 1983) cites losses of friendship, affordable possessions, self-worth, social and family status, identity, coherence and income, together with anxiety, insecurity, and the trauma of job-seeking from a disadvantaged position. While blue-collar workers are more likely to blame their unemployment on external factors, white collar workers lose the most in self-image and tend to blame themselves. Higher levels of depression were found to occur in women who were unemployed or married to unemployed men.

HEALTH AND SOCIOECONOMIC STATUS

Two decades ago, when poverty was rediscovered, in the midst of affluence, I wrote:

> Closer examination of the life-style of the poor has revealed that in nearly all aspects of health care, the poor behave and are treated differently from other sectors of the population.

We find that non-scientific health practices, fatalistic attitudes toward health, and the low ranking of medical care in the hierarchy of desirables are, together with the material disadvantages of the poor, impediments to the attainment of good health. (Paltiel, 1966, p. 33)

Data from a 1985 Canadian survey revealed that poor working women, while far more likely to have high blood pressure, were less likely to act to control this problem than nonpoor working women (Evalusearch, 1986). Moreover, when the same survey was analyzed on the basis of income only they found that:

The very poor were more likely to report high blood pressure and smoking than other income groups. In addition, obesity was most common among persons whose main activity was keeping house. High blood pressure, smoking, obesity and lack of exercise are risk factors for cardiovascular disease, so the data points to low-income women as having a number of characteristics placing them at risk. (Wilkins, 1986)

These results are corroborated by other Canadian studies that found cardiovascular risk factors to be higher among men and women with low education levels, and evidence that men and women in lower-socioeconomic groups are more likely to die from cardiovascular disease (Millar & Wigle, 1986).

The report *Alcohol in Canada* (Canada, 1984) suggests that while higher income groups are more likely to be current drinkers, lower-income drinkers are more likely to report alcohol problems.

The emerging picture suggests that the lowest-income groups are more likely to suffer negative effects of "risky" health behaviors than are their nonpoor counterparts. These "mal-adaptive" behaviors are not generally undertaken with a harmful intent, but they are coping behaviors (alcohol, drug or tobacco use) to provide comfort or relief from stressful lives. More effective, healthy, coping behavior might require an investment of time, energy, knowledge and money that is beyond the individual's or group's perceived or actual capacity (e.g., counselling, exercise, nutritious food, control or monitoring of health status).

Equally distressing is the admission in a recent textbook of psychiatry:

> In the past, long-term intensive, insight-oriented therapies usually have been reserved for intelligent, achievement-oriented patients with middle- or upper-class backgrounds and values. Psychotherapeutic approaches for lower-class patients have tended to be more authoritative, behavioral, supportive, symptomatic, short-term, and infrequent in nature, and usually combined with drugs. (Ludwig, 1978, p. 415)

STRESS

While work offers benefits it also entails risks. A review of the evidence associating stress with women's work roles, life conditions and social status follows.

Schuler (1984) defines institutional stress as a perceived dynamic state involving uncertainty about something important, e.g., opportunities, constraints or demands. The most salient definition is that of Lazarus and Cohen: "Stressors are demands that tax or exceed the resources of the system." The Dohrenwends (1984) also view stress as a transactional process between the individual and environment. Frankenhaeuser hypothesizes that psychologically arousing stimuli and events may lead to irreversible pathophysiological changes (1979). Epidemiological, life change and case studies suggest that stress is an important risk factor for a wide range of adverse health outcomes such as cardiovascular diseases, diabetes, gastrointestinal disturbances including ulcers and colitis, increased susceptibility to malignancies, infectious diseases and even death. All disease, particularly chronic illness, has its emotional concomitant.

Warshaw (1984) has called stress the most common toxic agent encountered in the workplace, affecting workers on all levels from the board room to the clean-up area, often in ways that are subtle, gradual and difficult to isolate. He sees it arising from the work itself, the way the work is organized, the physical and social environment, and/or relationships with superiors, peers and subordinates.

A five-community survey of Canadian Workers (CMHA 84) found that the opportunity to experience employment as a personally fulfilling activity appeared to be less available to women than to men. Women referred more often than men to structure and conditions of work and interpersonal relations on the job as sources of negative stress at work.

Occupational stress has been noted in connection with the high-speed assembly line, machine-paced work, rapid pacing, coercion, demands for sustained attention, monotony and repetition, overload and underload. Frankenhaeuser (1980) found that conditions characterized by uncertainty, unpredictability and lack of control usually produce a rise in adrenal output. Her data point to controllability as a major key to coping with distress. Since most women work under conditions in which they are subordinate to others, these three work conditions (uncertainty, unpredictability and lack of control) generally apply to large numbers of women (Paltiel, 1981).

Systematic studies of occupational stress in women are still scant and recent. The Framingham Study (Haynes & Feinleib, 1980) showed that among women, clerical workers were almost twice as likely to develop coronary heart disease (CHD) as either white- or blue-collar workers, and only among clerical workers were the rates of CHD greater in women than in men. Clerical workers with children, married to blue-collar workers, were more likely to develop CHD than nonclerical workers in the same situation. Moreover, clerical workers who developed CHD were likely to suppress hostility, to have a nonsupportive boss, to report fewer personal worries, and to experience fewer job changes.

Verbrugge (1984) comments that the Framingham study does not truly represent clerical workers since it included sales jobs. (The Framingham researchers have noted that they included mostly true clericals.) She argues further that the social milieu of the 1940s and 1950s when these women worked might explain their vulnerability. She suggests, without evidence, that contemporary clerical women probably have more pleasant and supportive work and home situations than the earlier decade, and hypothesizes that this reduces their risks of developing stress-related disease over the years. Yet the 1975-76 NHIS data she examined showed that both clerical women and men, when compared with other groups, were unsatisfied with their jobs. A Canadian Survey also confirmed that clerical workers least valued work for nonfinancial reasons (Canadian Mental Health Association, 1984).

A French study (Mamelle et al., 1984) which examined five categories of occupational fatigue factors in pregnant workers, i.e., posture, machine work, physical effort, mental stress and environment, found only two: mental stress and environment significantly increased the risk of pre-term delivery. Frankenhaeuser's (1978) research shows that the speed with which a person "unwinds" after stressful transactions with the environment will "influence the total wear and tear of the organism." Her study of female employees at an insurance company showed that after overtime work, even when the schedule was freely chosen, there was a spillover effect with pronounced elevation of adrenaline, elevated heart rate, as well as feelings of fatigue, noticed in the evenings under non-work condition at home. She has demonstrated experimentally that both underload and overload induce increased catecholamine secretion. Both induce stress and require effort. However, the uncertainty, unpredictability, and the lack of control that are associated with rise in output are reversed by confident task involvement.

Frankenhaeuser's experimental findings are supported by the National Institute for Occupational Safety and Health (NIOSH) studies, which suggest that the use of video display terminals (VDT) is not, in itself, a source of job stress, but that the stress was related to work activity (work load, work pace) and end result (goal). When clerical VDT users, clerical non-VDT users, and professional VDT users were compared it was found that clerical VDT users had no control over their work activity, the demands of the computer governing their work load and pace. This group showed the greatest stress. Non-VDT users having control over their work load and pace showed minimal stress, but were bored by their work activity, which had no goal (underload). Professional VDT users having a *goal* which utilized their education, experienced minimal stress (NIOSH, 1981).

In our accelerating high-tech, cybernetic society, we are discovering that the processes are using the persons rather than persons controlling the processes. Charlie Chaplin's "Modern Times" have indeed shifted from the factory to the office, with machine-yoked, machine-paced pink collar workers, minus the team work of the industrial assembly line. A recent survey of office workers (Stellman et al., 1984) found an association between higher-than-average levels of ergonomic stress due to workplace design problems and the incidence of musculoskeletal complaints at a site where a large number of the employees worked as VDT operators and sat in stationary positions for long periods every workday.

A U.S. National Survey on Working Women and Stress (9 to 5, 1984) also found that while higher level workers such as managers are more likely to describe their jobs as stressful, it is the lower level workers, such as clerks, who are more likely to experience stress-related health effects: eyestrain, headache, insomnia, muscle pain, fatigue, anxiety, anger and depression. The most stressful, damaging jobs were the ones combining high work demands with low control over the job (job strain).

Waldron has concluded that the effects of employment on women's health "vary, depending on the type of job and probably also on the family situation of the woman" (Waldron, 1983). She suggests that family responsibilities, time pressure, repetitive jobs and occupational hazards would contribute to adverse effects, while the reduction of these aspects along with social support and contact would lead to an increase in positive effects. Recognizing the "workplace" aspect of the home, she considers the social isolation and low status of the housewife role, but notes also that measures of psychological well-being which favor employed women of higher SES are not observed for women with less education and lower incomes.

Another large concentration of female workers occurs in the helping professions, with women extending their nurturant roles from the home to the workplace and in many cases straddling both. Elementary teachers, nurses, social workers and child care workers have high responsibility with low authority. Those who work mainly with the poor may be as overwhelmed as their clientele, while perceived by the latter as persons in authority and persons with power. Conflicts and powerlessness exact a price in mental health. Waldron (1978) notes that psychologists and female physicians have higher suicide rates than other women.

Burnout is defined by Maslach and Jackson (1981) as "a syndrome of emotional exhaustion and cynicism that occurs frequently among individuals who do 'people work' of some kind." While Pines (1978) defines burnout as " . . . a syndrome of physical and emotional exhaustion, involving the development of negative self-concept, negative job attitudes, and loss of concern and feeling for clients." The key aspect of burnout, namely emotional exhaustion, places burnout at the end of the spectrum of Selye's general adaptation or stress syndrome (1980). Burnout has been identified as a factor in job turnover, absenteeism, and low morale, correlated with self-reported indices of personal distress, including physical exhaustion, insomnia, increased use of alcohol and drugs, and marital and family problems. An important clue arising out of the studies on burnout is that it is associated with " . . . the belief that one's work is not very meaningful or worthwhile." However, once again feedback or knowledge of results appears to be a protective factor.

COPING

The growing field of stressology has been greatly influenced by Holmes and Rahe's Life Events (social readjustment) Scale (1967), originally comprised of 43 events. It measured the intensity and length of time necessary to accommodate to a life event, regardless of the desirability of this event, in contrast with Selye (1974), who distinguished between "good" (eustress) and "bad" (distress).

In discussing the life events stress research, Makosky (1982) notes the general lack of information about the effects of stress in women's lives. Sex comparisons were rarely reported, and the most frequently used lists of events included a disproportionate number of events which apply more often to men than to women, while excluding events which women are likely to experience. Thus being drafted, promoted at work, or having one's wife start work often appeared on inventories of stressful events, while experiencing an abortion, a rape, or a change in child care arrangements generally did not. In agreement with Brown and Harris, who discounted the additive life events approach, she notes that it is the steady, unchanging (or slowly changing) stressful life conditions which affect mental health. In Makosky's study of low-income mothers of young children she did not find that the number of life events was related to psychological well-being. The women at greatest risk for depressive symptoms, anxiety and poor self-esteem were the women "who had endured the most difficult stable conditions of life for the two years prior to the study." This also accords with the view of Fried (1982) that endemic stress is a condition of continuous and manifold changes, demands, threats or deprivations, frequently small in scale and embedded in daily life events.

The *Lives in Stress* study found that money was the strongest stress factor. Unpredictability, insecurity, and other problems associated with money were related to mental health, apart from the total amount of money available (Dill & Feld, 1982). Dill and Feld conclude that coping cannot be reduced to a single event in which a stressful stimulus calls forth a given response. They suggest that "difficulties low income mothers experience in coping lead to beliefs that they lack control over their environment and that their environment is unpredictable. These beliefs in turn erode the woman's motivation and sense of coherence" (p. 194). A curious finding of the *Lives in Stress* study was that contact with other adults was not a source of pleasure for the respondents. This was unexplained by the author but one hypothesis could be that these adults were not sources of support but sources of additional demands or stress. Indeed, Gore (1984) differentiates between continuing social support in chronic stress situations and support in crises, or life events, and challenges the support concept when it implies a characterization of social relationships as uniformly helpful and omits reference to the nonsupportiveness or indeed the hostility of some affiliates.

Commenting on the hypothesis that highly stressful events combined with low social support are significantly more pathogenic than highly stressful events with high social support, or less stressful events with high or low social support, Dohrenwend and Dohrenwend (1984) argue that such measures of social environmental conditions are probably also measuring level of personal competence in such a way that the two are positively associated.

The classic public health approach is the interactional effects of agent (the stressor), host, and environment. Miller (1980) and Lazarus tend to agree with the Dohrenwends about the role of perception and coping ability. The former contends that how one has learned to respond to a fear is frequently far more important than how afraid one is. Lazarus (1984) contends that what some perceive as a threat is viewed as a challenge by others. While environmental conditions themselves may provide a basis for this difference in cognitive appraisal, personality factors seem also to be important; some persons feel characteristically challenged, while others feel constantly threatened. That is why one cannot make dogmatic statements about poverty and mental health hazards.

Since threat and challenge may have different adaptational outcomes, this makes the distinction important. Lazarus suggests that those disposed to see demands in positive rather than threatening terms have two major advantages: higher morale, and the likelihood of better performance under pressure because they are more confident, less emotionally overwhelmed, and more capable of drawing upon their resources than those who are inhibited or blocked. The availability of resources, however, as well as problem solubility, remain as factors. Type A personalities who generally welcome challenges, set high standards and cope effectively with self-selected heavy work loads (Frankenhaeuser, 1978) are more prone to helplessness than controls when faced with uncontrollable events (Matthews & Glass, 1977).

Lazarus (1984) provides some clues to the coping styles of the poor and of women, by recognizing denial as a palliative form of coping. Denial, as a form of selective inattention or escapism, may be healthy in one context but life-threatening and risk-taking in another when it interferes with actions necessary to survival or constructive to change. Denial has been a life-threatening factor in wife battering ("It won't happen again, he didn't mean it") (Paltiel, 1982), while blaming the victim is a form of societal denial. One psychiatrist (Brill, 1977), for example, refers to Americans who "for some reasons have not been able to take part in the general social mobility to get themselves above the poverty level."

Frankl (1963), the founder of Logotherapy (a school of therapy based on insights gained from analyzing his and others' concentration camp experience), found clues to survival in "meaning in life" and survival for a purpose. "Existential frustration" he says, "is neither pathological nor pathogenic." Spiritual distress over the meaning of life is not mental disease and therefore should be not buried under a heap of tranquillizing drugs. (While I do not share Frankl's view that existential suffering is a necessary condition of humanity, I feel the greatest respect for those who have themselves undergone some transforming experiences which they interpreted as challenges.)

Antonovsky (1979) responding to Selye, has coined the term "salutogenesis" as a theory of "generalized resistance resources" to cope with stressors. His clue to coping and "salutogenesis" lies in a sense of coherence of individuals and groups, involving a perception of one's environment as predictable and comprehensible. The stronger the person's sense of coherence, he argues, the more adequately (s)he will cope with the imminent stressors in life, and the more likely (s)he is to maintain her/his position on the health ease/dis-ease continuum. Dimsdale (1976) and Caplan (1976) stress the intrapsychic personality factors associated with coping, such as mastery, focus on the good, trust in one's self, and basic optimism; but also acknowledge group affiliation and active invoking of help from others.

A MODEL FOR COPING

Seiden (1976) suggests that "Scientific revolutions are often at the beginning more conceptual than empirical; a new point of view often reorganizes old data before it stimulates the search for new data." One conceptual approach for policy development, based on the needs, risks and tasks of females and males in accordance with the life cycle and family cycle is presented here (see Figure 1). In this proposition, the mental health of adults of both sexes is dependent on three anchors—*work, family* and *friendship*. If the work anchor is absent or threatened, the adult can still function as (s)he can depend on the two remaining anchors, the family and friends. In cases of family breakdown, the adult who has work and friendship anchors intact may be sustained, compensated or reoriented during that breakdown. If

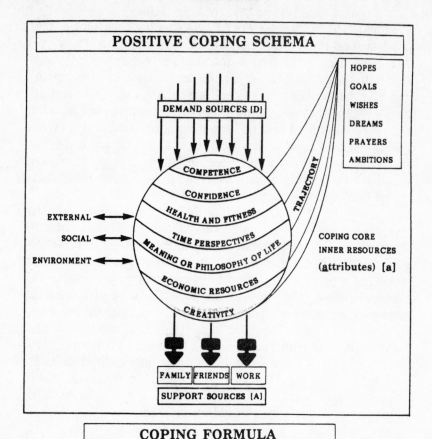

FIGURE 1

there is a breakdown in friendship, the anchors of work or family
may sustain the adult. Indeed, one may find compensatory companionship within the work or family situation when normal
friendship bonds have been severed and dislocated through geographic or social mobility. If one sustains loss of work and

friends and has or is expected to function with only one anchor, the family (as has been the normal situation for many married women), there is mounting evidence that this constitutes high risk for mild or moderate depression, particularly in isolated young women with children and in those middle-aged women whose full-time preoccupation has been care of the family.

The three-anchor-framework may be more useful for future-oriented research and policy formulation than the hierarchy of human needs, which places self-actualization on the highest plan. The framework posits a vision of society which is not a narcissistic utopia of autonomous individuals seeking to self-actualize. This is especially true since self-actualization has generally not applied to women, whose role-assignment has been the actualization of others, rendering them particularly vulnerable to domestic victimization and the handmaiden/supportive role in the workplace.

Seiden notes that both the need for companionship and the need for producing a tangible product are necessary in one's daily activities and that household maintenance does not fulfill these needs. She found that even when women were employed because of economic necessity, they still recovered from depression more quickly than housewives (Seiden, 1976).

The Canada Health Survey (1981), using two indicators of mental health, found that women are less happy and more prone to anxiety and depression than men. Women employed outside the home reported fewer negative feelings than women at home; however, a slightly higher proportion of women than men in the work force had "negative feelings." Unemployed women and those not in the labor force were more prone to anxiety and depression than were individuals who had jobs.

The Brown and Harris (1978) landmark studies on the social origins of depression concluded:

> The absence of an intimate tie or confiding relationship with a husband or boyfriend, the presence of three or more young children in the home and the loss of a mother before the age of 11 constitute the vulnerability factors. In addition, not having full or part-time employment outside the home is also a factor which, in the presence of a provoking agent, increases the risk. Working-class women have more of both

the vulnerability factors and the provoking agents. (Paltiel, 1980, p. 21)

In the model proposed here, the workaholic who neglects or abandons anchors of family and of friends is in a high-risk category, as is the single unattached individual, overly dependent on friendship without family or work. When two anchors are threatened, this signals high vulnerability and the need for therapeutic intervention. The highest risk of course is sustained when one lacks all three anchors: the unemployed, underemployed, single unattached individual in an impersonal metropolitan centre is clearly at risk for hopelessness and suicide (Langner & Michael, 1963). Conversely, good coping ability should occur in those adults, male and female, whose autonomous, yet interdependent and responsible lives are firmly anchored in work, friendship and family. The definition of family can begin with a conjugal pair, a mother and child, or an adoptive parent and child and places no limits on extensions that flow from these basic familial units, including the modern reconstituted family with all its branches (Paltiel, 1981).

Work is whatever a person defines as her or his work, whether left in or out of national accounts and statistics of "active" populations. However, good mental health, which involves self-esteem and the esteem of others, requires role congruence. It is better if there is a good fit between what persons call their work and that perceived as their work by others and rewarded as such.

The value and meaning of work to survival is perhaps most trenchantly expressed by Primo Levi: "One of the most important things I had learnt in Auschwitz was that one must always avoid being a nobody. All roads are closed to a person who appears useless, all are open to a person who has a function, even the most fatuous" (Levi, 1979). Being poor and a woman places one at terrible risk of being a nobody.

There even is a substantial body of data showing that animals given a choice between performing some operant response to earn food or accepting identical food freely available will choose to work for and earn the food. Commenting that this could be called "learned industriousness," Overmier (1980) interprets this as a preference for control, an important determinant of coping, indeed the flip side of Seligman's "learned helplessness"

(1975), the model of vulnerability to depression that accords so well with stereotyped sex-role expectations (Seiden, 1976).

CONCLUSION

Antonovsky, Lazarus and others have noted the importance of resources. These resources in sum are economic, social, psychological and biological. A fifth resource is time, often cited in relation to stress and pathogenesis, but seldom in relation to coping.

There is converging evidence from epidemiological and psychological studies for a "social support" hypothesis that mediates among the experience of stressors, life events, social conditions and the ability to cope. The model given here identifies the source of support as important. The fit between resources, supports and demands needs to be better understood, if we are to tailor our services to meet needs, identify and reduce hazards, and recognize and appreciate the tasks of women as family members, workers and citizens.

The author's proposed schema for positive coping and coping formula require testing and refinement. They are based on a three-anchor needs formulation plus a distillation of salient studies on stress and coping to provide direction and guidance for self-understanding and for helping women to acquire the resources, supports, attributes and perspectives to ensure that poverty at any time in their lives need not be an insistent, enduring, or inevitable threat to their mental health.

REFERENCES

Antonovsky, A. (1979). *Health, Stress, and Coping. In New Perspectives on Mental and Physical Well-Being.* New York: Jossey-Bass. (Cited in: F. L. Paltiel, Stress and Burnout in Women, 1981.)

Belle, D. (1982). Social ties and social support. In D. Belle (ed.), *Lives in Stress.* Beverly Hills: Sage.

Belle, D. et al. Mental health problems and their treatment. In D. Belle (ed.), *Lives in Stress, op cit.*

Boodoosingh, L. et al. (1986). The culturally deprived child.

Brill, N. Q. (1978). The problem of poverty and psychiatric treatment of the poor in the United States. *Psychiatric Journal of the University of Ottawa,* III, 3, 153-161.

Brown, G. W. & Harris, T. (1978). *Social Origins of Depression: A Study on Psychiatric Disorder in Women*. New York: Free Press. (Reviewed by F. L. Paltiel in Canada's Mental Health 28, 2, 1980.)

Buck, C. (1986). Beyond Lalonde: Creating Health. *Epidemiological Bulletin, PAHO*, 7, 2, 10-16.

Canada, Health and Welfare (1984). *Alcohol in Canada: A National Perspective*. Ottawa, Health and Welfare Canada.

Canada, Labour Canada (1986). *Women in the Labour Force*. Women's Bureau, Minister of Supply and Services Canada.

Canada, Statistics Canada (1984). *Income Distributions by Size in Canada*. Minister of Supply and Services Canada.

Canada, Statistics Canada (1985). *Women in Canada: A Statistical Report*. Minister of Supply and Services Canada.

Canada, Statistics Canada (1986). *Income distributions by size in Canada*. Statistics Canada.

Canada, Statistics Canada (1986). *The Labour Force Family Characteristics and Labour Force Activity: An Update*. Minister of Supply and Services Canada.

Canada, Health and Welfare (1986). *Evalusearch, Health Profiles of Four Labour Force Groups: Implications for Workplace*. Health and Welfare Canada.

Canada, Health and Welfare Canada (1986). *Progress Against Poverty*. National Council of Welfare.

Canada, Health and Welfare Canada (1986). The Pregnant Worker: A Resource Document for Health Professionals, prepared by the Federal/Provincial Working Group on the Development of Guidelines to Control Risks for Women in Industry to the Federal-Provincial Committee on Environmental and Occupational Health.

Canadian Mental Health Association (1984). *Work and Well-Being: The Changing Realities of Employment*. Canadian Mental Health Association, Toronto.

Canadian Mental Health Association (1983). *Unemployment: Its Impact on Body and Soul*, prepared by S. Kirsh.

Canadian Public Health Association (1981). Canadian Public Health Association, Edwards, P. (ed.), *Growing Together*. Ottawa.

Caplan, G. (1976). Human competence and coping. In *Human Adaptation: Coping with Life Crises*. Lexington: Heath and Co.

Dill, D. and Feld, E. (1982). The Challenge of Coping. In D. Belle (ed.), *Lives in Stress*, Beverly Hills: Sage.

Dimsdale, J. E. (1976). The coping behavior of Nazi concentration camp survivors. In R. H. Moos (ed.), *Human Adaptation: Coping with Life Crises,* Lexington: Heath and Co.

Dohrenwend, B. S. & Dohrenwend, B. P. (1984). Life stress and illness: Formulation of the Issues. In Dohrenwend, B. S. & Dohrenwend, B. P. (eds). *Stressful Life Events and their Contexts*. New Jersey: Rutgers University Press.

Economic Council of Canada (1983). *On the Mend*. Economic Council of Canada. Twentieth Annual Review.

Epp, J. (1986). Address of the Honorable Jake Epp, Opening Remarks — Scientific Session I — Health Related Behaviors *Canadian Journal of Public Health*, 77, Supp. 1, 5.

Frankenhaeuser, M. (1978). Psychoneuroendocrine approaches to the study of emotions as related to stress and coping. Nebraska Symposium on Motivation.

Frankenhaeuser, M. (1980). Psychoneuroendocrine Approaches to the Study of Stressful Person-Environment Transactions. In *Selye's Guide to Stress Research* 1. New York: Van Nostrand Reinhold.

Frankenhaeuser, M. (1980). Psychobiological Aspects of Life Stress. In S. Levin & H. Ursin (eds.), *Coping and Health*. New York: Plenum Press.

Frankl, V. E. (1963). *Man's Search for Meaning*. New York: Pocket Books.

Fried, M. (1982). Endemic stress: The psychology of resignation and the politics of scarcity. *American Journal of Orthopsychiatry*, 52, 1, 4-19.

Gore, S. (1984). Stress, buffering functions of social supports: An appraisal and clarification of research models. In Dorhnwend, B. S. & Dorhnwend, B. P. (eds.), *Stressful Life Events and their Contexts*. New Jersey: Rutgers University Press.

Haynes, S. & Feinleib, M. (1980). Women, work and coronary heart diseases: Prospective findings from the Framingham heart study. *Public Health*, 70, 2, 133-41.

Hollingshead, A. B. (1975). *Elmtown's Youth and Elmtown Revisited*. New York: John Wiley.

Hollingshead, A. B. & Redlich, F. C. (1958). *Social Class and Mental Illness: A Community Study*. New York: John Wiley.

Holmes, T. H. & Rahe, R. H. (1967). The social readjustment scale. *Journal of Psychosomatic Research*, 11, 213-218.

Langner, T. S. & Michael, S. T. (1963). *Life Stress and Mental Health*. London: Collier-MacMillan.

Lazarus, R. S. (1984). The costs and benefits of denial. In Dohrenwend, B. S. & Dohrenwend, B. P., (eds.), *Stressful Life Events and the Contexts*. New Jersey: Rutgers University Press.

Lazarus, R. S. et al. (1980). Psychological stress and adaptation: Some unresolved issues. In *Selye's Guide to Stress Research* 1. New York: Van Nostrand Reinhold.

Leighton, A. H. (1982). *Caring for Mentally Ill People: Psychological and Social Barriers in Historical Context*. Cambridge: Cambridge University Press.

Leighton, A. H. (1985). Poverty and social change. *Scientific American*, 212, 5.

Levi, P. (1979). *If This is a Man and the Truce*. Harmonsworth, NY: Penguin Books.

Liem J. H. & Liem R. (1984). Relations among social class, life events, and mental illness: a comment on findings and methods. In B. S. Dohrenwend & B. P. Dohrenwend (eds.), *Stressful Life Events and Their Contexts*. New Jersey: Rutgers University Press.

Ludwig, A. M. (1980). *Principles of Clinical Psychiatry*. New York: Free Press.

Mahler, H. (1985). Address to the Plenary Session of the World Conference. U. N. Decade for Women (Nairobi, 15-26 July). *Women and Health for All*: WHO Press.

Makosky, V. P. (1982). Sources of stress: Events or conditions? In Belle, D. (ed.), *Lives in Stress*. Beverly Hills: Sage.

Mamelle, N. (1984). Prematurity and occupational activity during pregnancy. *American Journal of Epidemiology*, 119, 3, 309-322.

Maslach, C. & Jackson, S. E. (1981). The measurement of experienced burnout. *Journal of Occupational Behavior*, 2, 2, 99-113. (Cited in F. L. Paltiel, *Stress and Burnout*, 1981.)

Matthews, K. A. and Glass, D. C. (1984). Type A Behavior, Stressful Life Events, and Coronary Heart Disease. In B. S. Dohrenwend & B. P. Dohrenwend (eds.), *Stressful Life Events and Their Contexts*. New Brunswick: Rutgers University Press.

Miller, N. E. (1980). Effects of learning on physical symptoms produced by psychological stress. In *Selye's Guide to Stress Research*, 1, New York: Van Nostrand Reinhold.

Millar, W. J. and Wigle, D. W. (1986). Socioeconomic disparities in risk factors for cardiovascular disease. *Canadian Medical Association Journal*, 134, 127-31.

Moffic, H. S. (1983). Attitudes in the provision of public sector health and mental health care. *Social Work in Health Care*, 8, 4, 18-28.

9 to 5 (1984). U. S. National Survey on Working Women and Stress.

NIOSH (1981). NIOSH National Institute of Occupational Safety and Health issues final VDT results, the newsletter of the International Word Processing Association, *Viewpoint*, 1, 4.

Overmier, J. B. et al. (1980). Environmental contingencies as sources of stress in animals. In S. Levine & H. Ursin (eds.), *Coping and Health*. New York: Plenum Press.

Paltiel, F. L. (1977). *New Frontiers in Mental Health*. A Report on a Pan American Health Organization/World Health Organization Fellowship.

Paltiel, F. L. (1966). *Poverty: An Annotated Bibliography and References*. The Canadian Welfare Council.

Paltiel, F. L. (1981). Shaping Futures for Women. *Women's Studies International Quarterly*, 4, 1, 13-25.

Paltiel, F. L. (1981). Stress and Burnout in Women, Notes for an Address to *W. O. H. R. C.* Conference, New York.

Paltiel, F. L. (1982). Women and pensions. *International Social Security Review*, 3, 1982, 333-344.

Paltiel. F. L. (1980). Vulnerability and critical stress points in women's life cycle. Paper presented at University of Western Ontario.

Pearlin, L. I. & Schooler, C. (1978). The structure of coping. *Journal of Health and Social Behavior*, 19, 1, 2-21.

Penfold, P. S. and Walker, G. A. (1983). *Women & the Psychiatric Paradox*. Montreal: Eden Press.

Pines, A. & Maslach, C. (1978). Characteristics of staff burnout in mental health settings. *Hospital and Community Psychiatry*, 29, 4, 233-237.

Sarwer-Foner, G. J. (1983). Phenomenology and natural course of the schizophrenia group of illness, diagnostic views and fashions in different countries. In Pichot, P. et al. (eds.), *Psychiatry: The State of the Art*. New York: Plenum Press.

Schuler, R. S. (1984). Organizational and occupational stress and coping: A model and overview. In Lee, M. D. & Kanungo, R. W. (eds.), *Management of Work and Personal Life: Problems and Opportunities*. New York: Praeger.

Seiden, A. M. (1976). Overview: Research on the psychology of women II. Women in families, work and psychotherapy. *The American Journal of Psychiatry*, 133, 10, 1111-1123.

Selye, M. (1980). *Selye's Guide to Stress Research*, 1, New York: Van Nostrand Reinhold.

Stavrakaki, C. (1985). Mental health of adolescents. *Proceedings of the Colloquium on Adolescent Girls' Health*, sponsored by the Office of the Senior Adviser, Status of Women, Health and Welfare Canada.

Stellman, J. M. et al. (1984). Occupational safety and health hazards and the psychosocial health and well-being of workers. In Cataldo, M. & Coates, T. (eds.), *Behavioral Medicine in Industry*. New York: John Wiley.

Verbrugge, L. M. (1984). Physical health of clerical workers in the U. S., Framingham and Detroit. *Women and Health*, 9, 1, 17-41.

Waldron, I. (1983). Employment and women's health: An analysis of casual relationships. In Fee, E. (ed.), *Women and Health: The Politics of Sex in Medicine*. New York: Baywood.

Waldron, I. et al. (1977). The coronary-prone behavior pattern in employed men and women. *Journal of Human Stress*, 3, 4, 2-18.

Warshaw, L. J. (1984). Occupational stress: What is it's significance. Paper presented at the American Occupational Health Conference, May.

Weitzman, L. J. (1985). *The Divorce Revolution: The Unexpected Social and Economic Consequences for Women and Children in America*. New York: Free Press.

Wilkins, R. W. (1985). Social Perspectives of Findings from the Canada Health Promotion Survey of 1985 (Draft). Paper prepared for Health and Welfare Canada: Montreal, August, 1985.

World Health Organization (WHO/Unicef) (1986). In Point of Fact, 34.

Afro-American Women, Poverty and Mental Health: A Social Essay

Maisha B. H. Bennett, PhD

SUMMARY. The experience of poverty can be a risk factor for mental illness. Afro-American women are disproportionately represented among the poor, the majority of whom are single mothers and heads of households who are concentrated in the secondary labor market and the secondary welfare system. These economic and social factors can engender stress and can limit opportunities for its resolution or for the gratification of psychological needs. The consequences can range from mild emotional distresses to severe mental illnesses. Recommendations for improving mental health status include public mental health promotion and education programs, and social, economic and political actions such as increased and better quality employment opportunities and educational system reforms.

Poverty is a risk factor for some forms of mental illness (see Paltiel, this volume). There is an unfortunate but strong and clear link between poverty status and a number of emotional and psychological disorders. This paper will focus on the experience of poverty for Afro-American women, the stresses engendered by poverty and the mental illness that can result when there is inadequate resolution of poverty-induced stresses.

Who are the poor? The poor are not a homogeneous group to be lumped together and ascribed a uniform set of characteristics (see Wilson, this volume). The poor include the unemployed,

Maisha B. H. Bennett, is Deputy Commissioner of Health, for Mental Health, Alcoholism and Substance Abuse, Chicago Department of Health, 50 West Washington Street, Daley Center, Room LL-139, Chicago, IL 60602.

low-wage earners, the elderly, the sick and disabled, one-parent families, and disproportionately, people of color. The poor are not merely individuals and families whose incomes fall below a certain level. Poverty is measured not only by income status, but also by financial resources, educational background, occupational skills, material possessions, and home environment. Poverty can also be a state of mind characterized by certain personal experiences, feelings and attitudes.

Just as Eskimo-Aleut languages include dozens of variations, nuances and connotations for the single English word "snow," so poverty in America is a concept with numerous variations. These variations are important to consider because they imply differential individual and group experiences with poverty-related stresses and a variety of strategies for coping.

Consider the concept of transient versus chronic poverty. An individual or family can suddenly or gradually become impoverished or one can have been born into poverty. The individual or family experiencing transient poverty will move out of poverty after some period of time, in some cases never again to experience poverty, and in other cases to experience poverty intermittently, continually moving back and forth from poverty to non-poverty status. For others, poverty may be chronic, with individuals or families remaining continuously for many, many years, if not forever in an impoverished state.

The experience of poverty is different for those raised in affluence who consciously and deliberately choose austerity compared with those raised in affluence who experience financial failures and thus become poor. And, both of these experiences are vastly different from those of people who are born into poverty because their parents were poor, as were perhaps their grandparents, their great-grandparents, and others before them. Such intergenerational poverty should be conceptualized differently from first-generation poverty.

Another concept is that of absolute poverty versus relative poverty. In absolute terms, if one's personal or family income falls below a certain level, one is classified as poor. But poverty is also relative, dependent on how financially well off an individual or family is compared to others in the community, in the country, in the world, in a particular ethnic group. An individual who is a low-wage earner living in a community where the majority of her neighbors are unemployed and/or on welfare is *relatively* better off than her neighbors. But when she leaves her community and sees how other people live, or reads national statistics, or watches television, she may find that she is considerably poorer than most other Americans. If she were to consider international data, however, she would find that her cash income, though possibly not her bargaining power, is greater than that of the majority of the population of a given impoverished country.

One can compare economic worth among members of ethnic groups in America. A low-wage earning white may be relatively poor compared to most other whites, while an Afro-American or Hispanic at that same low-income level may be relatively well-off compared to her ethnic peers. The low-wage earning white would probably be considered "poor" whereas the low-wage earning Afro-American may be considered "middle-income" compared to other Afro-Americans. Unlike the official classifications of poverty used by government agencies for various purposes, most Afro-Americans who are employed full-time and steadily would consider themselves (and would probably be considered by other Afro-Americans) to be "middle-class," paying much less regard to absolute income than to the educational level of the worker and the type of work done.

POVERTY AMONG AFRO-AMERICAN WOMEN

The Afro-American population was 26.5 million people in the 1980 census, with 35.6% of Afro-Americans living below the poverty level of $9,862 per year for a family of four, compared to 13% for the general population. Thus the rate for Afro-Americans was nearly three times that for whites.

The statistics that describe Afro-American women and poverty are quite alarming. Afro-American women are disproportionately represented among the poor, for particular reasons and with particular consequences. Pearce (1983) noted that,

Although the proportion of the poor who are Black did not change during the 1970's, the proportion who were in fam-

ilies headed by women increased. Indeed the decade of the
seventies saw a dramatic shift of the burden of poverty
among Blacks from male-headed to female-headed families. The number of Black families in poverty who were
maintained by men declined by 35%, while the number
maintained by women increased by 62%. In the course of
one decade, Black female-headed families increased from
about one-half to three-fourths of all poor Black families by
the 1980's.

In 1983, 47% of all Afro-American families were headed by
women, up from 8% in 1950 and 21% in 1960. Over half of all
Afro-American families that are headed by women have incomes
below the poverty level, compared to 30% for all female-headed
households and 7% for the nation's two-parent households.
Fifty-five percent of all Afro-American children are born to single mothers, many of them teenagers. In Chicago during 1983,
for example, 25% of all births were to teenagers and 95% of the
Afro-American teenagers who gave birth were unmarried. At the
same time, 49% of all Afro-American children in this country
lived in one-parent, female-headed households.

Two primary sources of support for Afro-American female-
headed households are the labor market and the welfare system.
In the labor market, Afro-American women are primarily concentrated in the secondary sector of a dual labor market (Pearce,
1983). (Primary-sector jobs are characterized by good pay,
fringe benefits, job security, unionization frequently, good working conditions, and due process in regards to job rights. Second-
ary-sector work is generally in marginal industries where jobs are
low-paying, often seasonal or sporadic, less likely to be union-
ized, and highly vulnerable to both economic trends and the idio-
syncracies of the employer.)

Within the welfare system, Afro-American women are concentrated in what can be considered a "secondary sector," if we
define "primary sector" welfare programs such as Social Security Retirement and Survivors Insurance (8.1% Afro-American
utilization), Medicare (9.3% Afro-American utilization), and
Veteran's compensation and pensions (10.0% Afro-American
utilization) as entitlement programs whose benefits are conferred

as a "right." Recipients of these benefits are not stigmatized, poverty is not an eligibility criteria, nor are degrading investigations of lifestyle required. Benefits are often more generous, and may not require the exhaustion of other resources. They may not be reduced in proportion to other income.

The "secondary welfare" sector, on the other hand, is characterized by low benefits, on the average, and eligibility criteria widely varied across states and even among localities within a state. These benefits are viewed as a privilege, not a right, can be revoked arbitrarily and for different reasons in different places, and are usually reduced in proportion to other income. Receipt of these benefits is usually stigmatizing both in the public's and in the recipients' perceptions. Secondary welfare sector benefits include Aid to Families with Dependent Children (34.2% Afro-American utilization), Food Stamps (34.2% Afro-American utilization), CETA public-service jobs (33.0% Afro-American utilization), Medicaid (34.9% Afro-American utilization), and Public Housing (36.0% Afro-American utilization). (These are also the benefit categories currently earmarked for the greatest federal budget cuts.)

HOUSEHOLD AND MARRIAGE STATUS

The phenomenon of impoverished Afro-American women suggests several themes, each with a set of psychological implications and consequences. Most Afro-American women who are poor are single. They are mothers and frequently young mothers. They are heads of households. Each of these circumstances can engender stress. If the circumstances are resolved positively or if there is adequate coping, then the woman can enjoy mental healthiness. If they are not resolved or if they are resolved negatively, she may experience emotional distress or even mental illness.

In 1980, 65% of Afro-American women ages 16 and over were single, including 34.4% never married, 8.7% separated, 9.1% divorced, and 12.8% widowed. These women manage their lives without the love, companionship and support that can be part of a conjugal relationship. Of course participating in a conjugal relationship will not guarantee love, companionship or support from an adult of the opposite sex, but not being in such a relationship will almost guarantee the absence of these conjugal emotional supports and benefits. Love, companionship and support are particularly important when there are children to be raised and a household to be managed and financed, especially in our complex society and difficult economic times.

Although women of all races both outlive and outnumber males in every age group, Afro-American male mortality rates are higher than those for any other sex-race group in this country, exacerbating the problem of male availability for Afro-American women. Afro-American males die at disproportionately higher rates from homicides, suicides, accidents and drug and alcohol-related causes. Nationally, there are 117 Afro-American women for every 100 Afro-American men. The ranks of eligible Afro-American males are further reduced by the disproportionately high percentages and large numbers of Afro-American men institutionalized in jails, prisons, detention centers and facilities for the mentally ill. The number of marriageable men is also reduced by those who are homosexual or asexual and those who are already "married" to alcohol or drug habits. The unemployed, those who do not consider themselves and/or are not considered by Afro-American women to be economically qualified for marriage, to be heads of household or even to be contributing members of households, further decrease the availability of suitable males.

COPING WITH BEING SINGLE

What are the stresses on an Afro-American woman that result from being single and from facing the realization that for her, as for many of the women around her, marriage is not a realistic option? How does she balance this reality against her need for conjugal love, companionship, sharing and support? How does this balance occur in a society in which marriage is considered the proper partnership, despite the widespread changes in social values and mores that have occurred and the drastic decrease in the percentage of Americans living in intact traditional families?

There are, of course, a variety of ways that impoverished

Afro-American women respond to being single. There are those who are single and celibate, who may engage in a number of church-related, family or community activities and feel that their lives are fulfilling. There are those who are single and celibate and feel miserable about themselves and their lives. There are unmarried women who, while single, have long-term, committed, and mutually supportive monogamous relationships with men. The majority of those who are single, however, do not have such relationships and are engaged in any of a wide variety of relationships with one or more men, either simultaneously or serially, either frequently or occasionally. The relationships may be intense or shallow, serious or casual. They may be mutually loving or exploitative. They may be brief or long-term, or there may be various permutations and combinations of all of the above.

CASE STUDIES: THE SINGLE WOMAN

Many poor women who are single experience feelings of isolation and loneliness that may eventually lead to depression, paranoia, anxiety disorders, substance use disorders, substance-induced organic mental disorders, and adjustment disorders. Their psychological needs for companionship, sharing, support or giving and receiving love are unmet because they are single and have not been able to establish consistent ongoing relationships and their poverty further reduces their options for achieving such relationships. Examples drawn from this author's clinical practice serve to illustrate these patterns.

Ayanna A. is a 42-year-old impoverished Afro-American woman who has never been married and has no children. She came into therapy for the treatment of anxiety and depression. It was found that her psychiatric symptoms were closely related to the difficulties she was having establishing and maintaining heterosexual relationships. Although her history included several long-term relationships, they alternated with long periods of celibacy. She demonstrated low self-esteem and little self-confidence with men, particularly if they were her intellectual peers. Although Ayanna

intensely desired the emotional intimacy and support she
knew could be possible with a man, she was fearful of let-
ting any man get close to her or really know her. She was
equally fearful that with the scarcity of men, even if she
opened herself to a relationship, no man would respond to
her. Ayanna continues in therapy, presently trying to resolve certain psychological issues so that she can gather the
courage to safely and healthfully end three and one-half
years of celibacy and engage in a satisfying relationship.

Motherhood and Poverty

The stresses of being single are exacerbated by the stresses of
motherhood. Motherhood is a role that is complex and demand-
ing, even under the best economic and social conditions. The
difficulty is increased for poor women with limitations on both
financial and social resources. How does an Afro-American poor
woman meet the responsibility of raising children to be well-
adjusted, productive, and successful (even happy) adults with
limited resources? How does she balance out the demands of
mothering children with her own personal psychological needs
for achievement, for affiliation, for happiness? The situation for
adolescent mothers is even more complex because adolescents
are still struggling to make their own full psychological transition
from childhood to adulthood. And the woman who finds that she
is not happy with or suited to this role generally cannot change
her mind without incurring severe societal disapproval. As the
demands, the responsibilities, the stresses and the strains of
motherhood become overwhelming, they can damage both
mother and child, resulting in child abuse and neglect that can
range from physical assault to verbal assault, which though more
subtle may be no less damaging. The mother can suffer from
depression, anxiety, personality disorders and other chronic
stress-related disorders.

Motherhood contains the potential for immense joy and satisfaction. Full and successful execution of the mother's role can
promote the greatest actualization of the human potential. A
woman can reach into the depths of self-knowledge through
knowing her child. She can reach the heights of personal growth

and character development through loving him unconditionally and giving to him unselfishly. She can expand the breadth of her soul through nourishing his soul. If a mother is overwhelmed by poverty, by too many needs and too few resources, by too many problems and too few solutions, motherhood can become one of the greatest failures and sources of self-doubt and low self-esteem that a woman can experience. The experiences of Carla are illustrative.

Carla S. is a 32-year-old Afro-American mother of five. After becoming pregnant with her first child at age 17, she married the baby's father. Two years later they had a second child. The marriage ended with a separation after five years and eventual divorce six years later. Soon after separating from her husband, Carla began to live off and on for the next ten years with another man, Charles. This man has fathered two of her children. During one period of separation from Charles, Carla married an Arab immigrant. She reportedly married for love, and he apparently for citizenship because he deserted Carla the day after his citizenship became final. During a recent separation from Charles, Carla became pregnant and bore her fifth child. She claims not to be sure of the paternity of this child because she was dating several men at the time she became pregnant.

Carla has supported her family alternately through public assistance benefits and through a low-paying job as a hospital laboratory assistant. She has also supplemented her income with money given to her by Charles from his disability benefits.

Carla presented herself for therapy because she was having great difficulty managing her children. When she was employed she always worked the night shift so that she would be at work while the children were sleeping. She generally spent the afternoons and evenings locked in her room away from the children, leaving them on their own, ostensibly to get sleep to prepare to go to work. Carla was at a loss as to how to handle the oldest child, a daughter, who became openly sexually active at age eleven. She did not know what to say to her daughter about her sexuality or about birth control. When Carla's second daughter turned eleven and began to show signs of interest in sex, Carla asked the therapist to talk with her daughter, expressing doubts about her own abilities to provide the "right answers" or to be an appropriate role model in light of her own marriage and child-bearing history. Her third and fourth children, a boy and a girl, both preadolescent, exhibited behavior problems at home and at school. They were uncontrollable, disobedient, argumentative, and pugnacious. Carla had totally given up any hope of managing these two children.

Carla was diagnosed as suffering from bipolar disorder and depression. She was most frequently in a depressed state characterized by hopelessness, irritability, hypersomnia, fatigue, and guilt, alternating occasionally with periods of expansiveness and physical restlessness.

Managing Household Responsibilities

"Head of household" is a term that connotes "primary responsibility for the welfare and well-being of the members of that household." In our society, the family unit is responsible for its members in a number of areas. It is the family that is primarily responsible for supplying the basics of food, shelter and clothing; emotional support, sharing, caring and love; the development and maintenance of morality, values, and ethics; the transmission of history, culture and traditions; sex-role identity and gender-appropriate behaviors; male-female relationship skills; interpersonal skills; problem-solving skills; health maintenance; and protection and safety. The head of household is traditionally charged with responsibility for ensuring that these duties are discharged.

Many of these responsibilities, such as the provision of food, shelter and clothing, are difficult if not impossible for the poor, single, female head of household. When one is poor, one's income is consistently considerably less than one's expenses. No amount of juggling or thrift will make the budget balance.

Poor, single, Afro-American mothers include those who work, primarily in the secondary labor market (see Stellman, this issue); those who receive government assistance, primarily in the "secondary welfare" system; and those who try to supplement their meager wages with welfare benefits, or supplement their meager welfare benefits with wages (frequently in violation of government regulations). The total welfare allocation per family in many states, including Illinois, is approximately 50% of the income that is considered to be at the poverty level. Annual income for a family of four of $9,780 or below is defined as poverty, but annual government welfare payments to a mother and three children can be less than $4,400 in many areas. Thus the mother starts out with a deficit budget. How does she provide even the basics of food, shelter and clothing for her family? Many poor, single mothers who are heads of their households expend tremendous energy worrying, scheming and praying about how to make ends meet.

Poor women have been forced to be creative in attempts to supplement their incomes. Many women seek contributions of money, food, clothes and gifts from boyfriends, lovers, or casual sexual liaisons. A few depend to some extent on income from illegal activities such as prostitution, drug sales and the like. The case studies on Carla and Sandra serve as examples.

> During the course of therapy, Carla S. struggled with the dilemma of whether to renew her relationship with the father of her two oldest children, a man who flaunted his other girlfriends before her, and who never helped her financially, but whom she felt she loved. Or, should she reunite with the father of her second set of children, a man who was possessive and argumentative but who freely gave her money to help with household expenses?

> Sandra T., another poor, Afro-American, single parent, stated in therapy that she made ends meet financially by taking the bus from Chicago to Detroit one weekend per month in order to "turn tricks."

The struggle for economic survival results in intense, continuous and unabating stress on the poor, female head of household. For many poor, Afro-American, single female heads of household, poverty is perpetual. Such chronic, unmitigated and unresolved stresses can lead to serious emotional distress and possi-

bly to mental illness. In addition, many of these mothers, unable
to execute their responsibilities successfully, are losing their children to gangs, drugs, alcohol, violence, teenage sex and consequent pregnancies. Although the causes of such phenomena are
complex and related to social, economic, political and psychological conditions and not necessarily the mother's "fault," the
head of household role implies a responsibility to guide one's
children to the best of one's ability through the maze of childhood and adolescence safely to adulthood. Thus *ipso facto* the
female head of household can be considered to have failed in this
role.

The mother herself may also be suffering from limited positive
life experiences and few experiences with success, a legacy of
poverty, limited visions of future possibilities for her children,
deficiencies in being able to serve as a role model, difficulty
providing positive male role models, personality disorders, emotional distresses such as depression or anxiety, and limitations in
providing housing for the family in more wholesome neighbor-
hoods. All of these add to the difficulty, even impossibility of her
role.

Can an impoverished, single, female head of household teach
her children good male-female relationship skills or gender-appropriate behaviors? It is difficult because much of this learning
takes place as children witness the dialectic between their fathers
and their mothers and learn from their parents as role models.
Can she provide emotional support for her family? Again, this is
formidable because, for many women who are emotionally
drained by the demands of single parenthood and getting few of
their own emotional needs met, there is often not enough in their
emotional reservoir to give as fully and freely as each child requires.

It should be fully acknowledged that there are some success
stories among impoverished, single mothers who are heads of
household. There are some women who not only manage as
mother and as head of household, but who also create for themselves happiness, satisfaction and success. These women are
psychologically well-balanced and free from major emotional
distress or mental illness.

On the other hand, for some women the experience of motherhood as head of the household feels like failure, particularly if she compares her lot to that of other women who are economically more advantaged. She may then feel lowered self-esteem, dejection, hopelessness, anger, resentment, depression and other negative emotions. Poor resolution of these feelings could lead to diagnosable emotional distress.

Those women who are second or third or more generation impoverished have more likely than not inherited a "legacy of poverty," including a set of poverty-perpetuating attitudes and behaviors characteristic of poor people that, in turn, reinforce and perpetuate poverty status by decreasing the likelihood of purposeful behavior geared toward escape from poverty. Women chronically impoverished may become fully submerged in a "culture of poverty." Afro-American women have been found to have less likelihood of escape through marriage or through employment. There is a great "shared fantasy" among poor people that their primary, perhaps only hope of escape from poverty is through winning the lottery. Unfortunately, it is true that for many the odds of escaping poverty are about as slim as the odds of winning the lottery.

Positive and Negative Coping

Healthy resolution of stressful life circumstances is accomplished by adaptive coping and can lead to good mental health. Poor or inadequate resolution can lead to emotional distresses and even mental illness. Many impoverished Afro-Americans seek to escape feelings of depression and hopelessness by drinking. They may use alcohol to try to forget the pain of trying to survive from day to day. As a result, many lose control of their drinking and become alcoholics. The following is a clinical example.

Ms. K. is a 36-year-old mother of four children, single and unemployed. She is a second generation public-housing dweller and recipient of public aid benefits. Her childhood years were filled with just the bare necessities. She started drinking as a teenager to cope with the embarrassment of not being able to dress like her peers. She dropped out of school without any marketable skills and tried to obtain employment. Failing to get a job, she then drank to help cope with her idle time. When she became a single parent, she drank more to cope with parental responsibilities. She had some periods of sobriety while in a government job-training program, but returned to heavy drinking when this program was eliminated. Her daily use of alcohol caused her to neglect her children. Her neighbors reported the situation to the Department of Children and Family Services, which threatened to take her children if she did not seek treatment for her alcoholism. Fearing the loss of both her children and her source of income, she entered treatment for her alcoholism. However, her prognosis for sobriety is poor based on her inability to change her environment and on her pessimism about improving her lifestyle.

RECOMMENDATIONS

When a situation is as difficult and complex as the mental health status of impoverished, Afro-American women, recommendations for addressing the situation are equally difficult and complex. While serious, the situation is by no means hopeless.

The first recommendation is for extensive public mental health promotion and education programs and campaigns geared toward changing attitudes and behaviors among the poor that reinforce and perpetuate their poverty. Such efforts are particularly important for the multi-generational poor and the chronically poor. In order to be effective, such programs must be started as early in life as possible. The development of values, attitudes and approaches to solving life's problems begins when life begins and there appear to be certain critical developmental years when a child crystallizes much of the kind of person she will be and the way she will approach life. However, public mental health promotion campaigns geared toward breaking the cycle of poverty must be continued throughout adulthood, as every human being, no matter what age, retains the potential for growth and change.

Mental health could be promoted by programs conveying several messages that might be internalized by people. The messages could aim at helping people regularly take stock of themselves: who they are and where they want their lives to go. Most people could benefit from an honest appraisal of the attitudes and behaviors that are *truly* in their own best interests and that will help them achieve the life goals they desire. Most of the behaviors that a person engages in, even those that appear negative or destructive, are chosen because the individual perceives that one or more of her needs or self-interests are being served by that behavior. For example, drugs may give her pleasure, gang activities may boost her self-esteem or give her a sense of power, teenage sexuality may provide her with feelings of intimacy and the sense that somebody really cares. So the challenge for public mental health promotion becomes one of weighing out and eliminating attitudes and behaviors that may provide immediate, though temporary and in many cases, illusionary gratification and towards adopting attitudes and behaviors that promote one's true self-interests.

This is no easy task. Not only does it require frequent and continual reassessments, but it also requires enough self-love and self-esteem to actually do what is in one's own best interest. Further, to be successful, one must develop and utilize a repertoire of alternative healthy attitudes and behaviors that are incompatible with the perpetuation of poverty. A public mental health promotion program that can interrupt the cycle of poverty, for some people at least, will strengthen personality characteristics that can facilitate an individual's exit from poverty, will help individuals understand and choose attitudes and behaviors that are in their own best self-interests, and will increase self-esteem to the level where people care enough about themselves to be good to themselves.

Although mental health promotion campaigns can be effective for a segment of the population of impoverished Afro-American women, such programs will not solve the problem for all. Poverty is a social and political problem as well as an economic problem. Therefore, political, social and economic actions will be required to reduce or eliminate poverty and thus reduce or eliminate consequent psychological problems.

There are a number of areas related to poverty where social, political and economic changes are important. The most obvious is employment. The poor need more opportunities for employment. There are not enough jobs for all the people who want to work. Jobs that currently fall in the secondary sector of the labor market need to more closely approximate primary sector jobs in terms of an adequate minimum wage standard, fringe benefits, and job protection. Another obvious area is the need for reforms in the welfare system to make benefits more realistic and more conducive to family stability and integrity and to the presence of husbands and fathers. The educational system needs reform so that students learn to reason, to be healthy, and to prepare for meaningful futures. Political, social and economic changes will require action on the part of the poor and other individuals and organizations who care about justice and freedom for all people.

Poverty can be a risk factor for mental illness. But the risks can be significantly reduced by public mental health programs and by political, social and economic actions that impact on the current systems that perpetuate poverty.

REFERENCES

Bennett, Maisha B.H. (1979). Black children: Handle with care. *Black Child Journal, I* (1).

Holman, Robert (1978). *Poverty: Explanations of Social Deprivation.* New York: St. Martin's Press.

Luft, Harold S. (1978). *Poverty and Health.* Cambridge, Mass.: Ballinger Publishing Co.

Pearce, Diana M. (1983, Nov/Dec). The Feminization of Ghetto Poverty. *Society.*

U.S. Department of Commerce, Bureau of the Census (1983, 1984). *Detailed population characteristics. United States summary*, Volume 1, Chapters B-D.

Poverty, Self-Concept, and Health: Experience of Latinas

Carlota Texidor del Portillo, EdD

SUMMARY. America's largest minority group at the beginning of the twenty-first century will be Hispanics/Latinos. Only a few years away from the new century, this group faces the sad reality of being at the lowest rung of the economic ladder, exhibiting poor health, being ignored in the data-collection process, and thought of as having low self-concept.

A brief review of who they are and a summary of the data available in the areas of poverty, self concept, and health as they pertain to Hispanas/Latinas are provided. (The term "Hispanic" and "Latino" will be used interchangeably to describe the same population.) A vocational and counseling approach used at San Francisco Mission Community College is described and its effectiveness for Hispanic women is discussed. Recommendations for future work are provided.

BACKGROUND

The term "Hispanic" does not define a race, ethnic group, or nationality. Neither is it the term of choice in Latino districts. Rather, it is a convenient and bureaucratic catch-all to describe immigrants to the United States and their descendants from more than thirty countries in which the Spanish language is spoken. As such, it masks much diversity. The three largest groups of Hispanics—Mexican-Americans, Puerto Ricans, and Cuban-Americans—comprise 80 percent of the Latino population in this nation. Mexican-Americans are by far the largest subgroup, accounting for about 60 percent of Hispanics in this country and

Carlota Texidor del Portillo is Director of Student Services, Center's Division, San Francisco Mission Community College, 106 Bartlett Street, San Francisco, CA 94110.

229

concentrated in a crescent from Texas to California. Puerto Ricans represent 14 percent and are centered in the eastern U.S. They seem to be on the lowest rung of the Hispanic economic ladder, having the largest proportion of households headed by women, the highest school dropout rate, and the lowest income of all Hispanic groups (U.S. Bureau of the Census, 1982). Cuban-Americans account for 6 percent of the Hispanic population and represent the economic elite. The first two waves of those who fled Castro's Cuba were professionals and businessmen; many were affluent. The remaining 20 percent that make up the Hispanic population of the United States are comprised of people from Central and South America who live throughout the urban centers of the United States.

Similarities in culture and a common language bind the different groups. For the transplanted Latino, language maintenance has become a critical social and educational issue as well as a symbolic affirmation of worthiness (Taylor, 1984). National diversity and the social cleavages reproduced from the country of origin, however, help to keep them divided.

On the strength of fertility alone, Latinos will supplant all other minorities as the nation's most populous minority group early in the next century. Adding to the growth in the number of Latinos in the U.S. are about 600,000 Hispanic immigrants who have been arriving annually since the late 1970s. This trend is likely to continue as political unrest and economic conditions worsen in Spanish-speaking countries (Taylor, 1984).

There are significant demographic differences between Hispanics in this country. In 1985 the median age of Hispanics was 25 years, compared with 31.9 years for the non-Hispanic population. Median Hispanic family income in 1984 was $18,800 compared to $27,000 for non-Hispanics (U.S. Bureau of the Census, 1982).

Most Latino immigrants are economically disadvantaged and the migratory experience of these impoverished immigrants place them at the bottom of the socioeconomic heap. Employment attained immediately after migration often represents a step down from the jobs left in the society of origin (Rogler, 1983). Until recently, Hispanics have been an "invisible" minority largely unaffected by affirmative action policies. Discrimination has had serious consequences on the economic well-being of Latinos and has excluded many from the mainstream of U.S. society. The average unemployment rate for Hispanics in 1983 was 13.8 percent compared to 8.4 percent for whites (Ford Foundation, 1984). In 1982, nearly 30 percent of Hispanic families lived in poverty, two-and-a-half times the proportion for whites. Economic mobility is slow as well. Poor education and employment discrimination combine to keep large numbers of second-generation Latinos from achieving economic security.

For Latinas, the economic picture is even worse. The data generally show that the income of Latinas is inadequate to meet standard living needs and much lower in comparison with the incomes of other groups of women. In 1982, Hispanic women reported the lowest income of any racial-ethnic group, 9.5 percent lower than that reported for Anglo females (California Commission on the Status of Women, 1983).

If education is indeed a prerequisite for economic self-sufficiency, statistics on Hispanic educational preparation and attainment are sources of real concern. Hispanics have high dropout and illiteracy rates coupled with below-grade-level school enrollment. The overall Hispanic dropout rate stands at 37 percent, though some research puts this figure much higher. For Hispanics who remain in school, they are less likely to earn top grades and almost two-thirds are enrolled in vocational education programs that make college improbable if not impossible. Furthermore, Hispanic teachers are dramatically underrepresented in the teaching force, one factor cited by dropouts for leaving school. A report issued recently by the National Council of La Raza concludes that improving the education of the growing numbers of minorities is a national imperative in that it is in the nation's economic and political interests to do so (National School Public Relations Association, 1986).

Another indicator of poor educational achievement is the relatively low number of Hispanics enrolled in graduate schools. In 1976-77 there were 20,274 Hispanics in the U.S. attending graduate schools, increasing to 24,402 in 1984-85 (*The Wall Street Journal,* 1986). While this represents a 20.4 percent increase in Hispanic enrollment in graduate schools over the intervening eight years, an enrollment of 24,402 represents a mere .0014 percent of a total population of 17 million Hispanics.

The U.S. is home for the sixth largest Hispanic population in the world, 16.9 million men, women and children, and the numbers are expected to double every five years. Yet policy-relevant knowledge of the Hispanic population is still severely lacking (Ford Foundation, 1984). Federal policymakers have little data to draw on for assessing the health and nutritional status of Latinos, determining the needs and priorities for health care, and analyzing the relationships between health outcomes and risk factors. For example, when Margaret M. Heckler was appointed Secretary of the U.S. Department of Health and Human Services (HHS) in 1983, she expected to find a wealth of data on the health problems and progress of Hispanics in this country. Instead, she found a vast information gap. HHS staff had no information on the number of Hispanics who die in a given year, much less specific data that could assist them in isolating specific health factors that increase mortality rates among Hispanics (Heckler, 1985). This abysmal lack of information impedes the development of informed federal social and health policies.

HEALTH

The limited information on Hispanic health issues is cause for concern. In 1984, the National Center for Health Statistics conducted the National Health and Nutrition Examination Survey (NHANES). The sample of Hispanics, however, was too small to make meaningful statements about Hispanics as a whole or to make valid comparisons with other groups (Heckler, 1985). The Hispanic Health and Nutrition Examination Survey (HHANES) was subsequently undertaken to fill this void. HHANES was designed to provide estimates of the health and nutritional status for the Mexican-American, Cuban-American, and Puerto Rican that are comparable to those available for the general population (U.S. Department of Health and Human Services, 1985). The analyses of these data will help shed light on the state of health among Hispanics, but it will be incomplete as it will not provide information on the other Hispanic groups.

From the small sample of Hispanics surveyed under NHANES,

valuable information was produced in one area — the scope of the medically uninsured. Twenty-six percent of the Hispanics surveyed were found to have no health insurance coverage, compared to 18 percent for blacks and 9 percent for whites. Mexican-Americans were the group with the highest proportion uninsured — almost one in three (Heckler, 1985).

Many problems, such as air pollution, sexually transmitted diseases, and malnutrition affect the poor more than the affluent. As Hispanics are over-represented in the lower economic levels of the society, one can infer that these problems will affect them in a disproportionate manner. In fact, Hispanic women make up a substantial part of the low-wage labor force in some areas of this nation. The small factories and shops from Los Angeles to Chicago and from Houston to New York continue to employ Hispanic women at the lowest wages in the land. Hispanic women also labor at harvesting crops in California, Arizona, and Texas where the safety level of hazardous pesticides is under dispute. Their health and that of their families suffer as a direct result of this exploitation.

Since comprehensive data on the health of Latino women are not available, we are left to glean bits of information from the few observations that have been reported. Castellanos (1985) reports that Hispanic women are undertreated for post-menopausal syndrome along with its multitude of related conditions. In addition, menopause, depression, and several "psychosomatic" complaints are conditions commonly misunderstood and misdiagnosed.

Pietro (1985) reports that in his many years of practicing medicine, he has observed a pattern in the help-seeking behaviors of Hispanic women in the U.S.: they seek care only when a critical need is present. Quality care is generally too expensive, fragmented, and technologically impersonal for them as well as for their families to seek treatment sooner.

MENTAL HEALTH

A person's economic status and physical health have been long recognized as affecting mental health. The mentally healthy enjoy the fullest benefit of their capabilities and avoid preventable harm to themselves and others. Most often, mental health is manifested by an individual's expression of well-being. The basic conditions of well-being include economic stability, adequacy of income, good health and a positive self-concept, enabling the individual to be socially effective and to participate in the society at large. People living in poverty do not enjoy the material and the psychological components associated with well-being. The data on Hispanics seem to indicate that this group is at high risk and likely to suffer from poor mental health.

The important issue of mental health among Hispanics has been affected by flawed and disparate research (Rogler, 1983). Rogler (1983) reaffirms the lack of reliable epidemiological data on the incidence and prevalence of psychological distress in the Hispanic populations. The Report to the President's Commission on Mental Health (1978) states that

> . . . quality has not kept pace with quantity and the research literature on Hispanic mental health has yet to attain the status of an integrated body of scientific knowledge. It remains plagued by stereotypic interpretations, weak methodological and data-analytic techniques, lack of replicability of findings and the absence of programmatic research. (Special Populations Sub-Task Panel on Mental Health of Hispanic Americans, 1978)

In the absence of well-designed community-based epidemiological research that disentangles important sources of error, the case for high rates of psychological distress among Hispanics rests largely upon inferential evidence (Rogler, 1983).

Hispanics underutilize mental health services in relation to their mental health needs. They are prone to be misdiagnosed because of culturally insensitive diagnostic procedures. The treatment they receive typically does not fit their culture and life circumstances. And, they often experience difficulty in resuming customary social roles after undergoing treatment (Rogler, 1983).

There is some evidence that Hispanic women in the U.S. are a group at high risk of developing mental illness (Becerra, 1982).

Depressed socioeconomic conditions as well as role conflicts experienced as a result of migration and acculturation contribute to placing Hispanic women at risk (Canino, 1982). The research describing the diagnoses of Hispanic women indicates that depression and psychosomatic disorders are frequent among this population. Of the many mental ills affecting Latinos, depression is the most commonly cited condition. *Hispanic Mental Health Research* (Newton, Olmedo & Padilla, 1982), a reference guide, describes 31 studies on Hispanics and depression. Cognitive theorists propose that depression results from the development of maladaptive attitudes, over-reaction to specific stresses, and traumatic events. Cognitive manifestations of depression include low self-esteem, hopelessness, and helplessness (Baskin, 1981). Information is not available, however, to make definitive statements about the prevalence of these disorders among Hispanic women. Neither do we have the data to determine whether these indices of poor mental health are idiosyncratic to culture or to social class (Bercerra, 1982).

Cultural demands have imposed upon the Latino woman a self-denying, self-sacrificing role in which she cherishes her children and husband but asks very little for herself (Gibson, 1975). Gibson claims that Latino women must change their roles and self-concept if they are to partake of the advantages of modern society. Llanes (1975) claims that the Latina's self-effacing role fits well within her culture but renders her dysfunctional under certain conditions in the American society. In short, the Latina is expected to be submissive and self-denying and this behavior is rewarded with extensive praise. This fits well into the theory that an individual's expectancy for reinforcement is related to social role and to perceptions of the forces that control one's life. When the male provider and the environment that reinforces her submissive role are absent, however, the Latina becomes dysfunctional.

Addressing the mental health needs of this population can be a monumental task in the absence of a strong, unified body of research and developed practices. Individual practitioners are left to their own resourcefulness to implement programs that address the needs of Latinas caught up in a cycle of poverty, poor health, and ineffectiveness. From mental health practitioners serving the Hispanic population are reports that Hispanic patients often do not respond to traditional, psychodynamic, insight-oriented psychotherapies (Torres-Matrullo, 1982). There appears to be some agreement among clinicians concerning the applicability and effectiveness of more structured, goal-oriented behavioral approaches when working with Hispanic patients, particularly those who are not psychologically minded and those from lower socioeconomic backgrounds.

Miranda (1976) reports that when Hispanics enter mental health clinics they expect treatment to be characterized by immediate symptom relief; guidance and counseling; a concrete focus; a problem-centered approach; and responsiveness, cultural sensitivity and reliability on the part of the therapist. Literature is available on implementing behavioral and structured treatment models for Spanish-speaking populations (Miranda, 1976). Because the cognitive behavioral approach is structured and goal-oriented, Torres-Matrullo (1982) reports the suitability of this approach in treating Puerto Rican women.

OBSERVATIONS AT SAN FRANCISCO MISSION COMMUNITY COLLEGE

There is a scarcity of studies focusing on the mental health needs of Latino women. What is becoming evident, however, is that the Latino woman comprises a unique at-risk group. She is affected by the role imposed upon her by her culture. She is disproportionately affected by the prevailing conditions of the society at large and by a number of personal conditions brought about by a poor educational background, the quality of her health care, and a projected poor self-concept when assessed by the U.S. culture. Because of the lack of an integrated research literature, practitioners working with Latinas often must improvise strategies that address their clients' needs in a practical and culturally relevant manner.

In working with women at San Francisco Mission Community College Center, this writer and the counseling staff often found it both frustrating and counterproductive to carry on intensive counseling and to focus on a problem only to discover the client incapable of taking the next step to resolving that problem. Several factors were difficult to overcome, such as undereducation, lack of job skills, disorientation to the majority culture, lack of uncommitted funds, and an absence of family support for the women's goals, inability to speak English well, religious dogma, inflexible role expectations as well as family obligations. Far more counterproductive, however, was the pervasive fear to contemplate success. The women claimed that they were not satisfied with their lives but did not welcome changes that would produce conflict with family members or friends.

An effective strategy that would pull these women out of the marasmus in which they existed was needed. A counseling approach needed to be developed that would enable the counselor to convincingly demonstrate the client's ability to succeed so that the women would begin to believe in their own ability to succeed and also begin to act in ways reflecting this new perception.

Based on the theory that action precedes attitude, a study carried out at San Francisco Mission Community College Center examined and demonstrated the effectiveness of minimal success therapies on positive attitudinal change among Latino women (del Portillo, 1980). It also reported that minimum success strategies in job-related areas altered the self-concept of Latino women and that positive changes became evident in job interviews. Based upon 15 years of experience counseling Latino women as well as developing and implementing curricula for vocational programs to meet their needs, this author concludes that intervention strategies that alter the emotional state of dysfunctional Latinas must become a priority of our communities.

Among hundreds of Latinas who have been interviewed or counseled at San Francisco Mission Community College Center (an adult education center), the prevalent and most often-expressed desire was to learn the way to economic success. These women wished to change their economic status as the primary step toward solving the problems in their lives.

It has been our observation that, in every case, a short-term goal that had been set and realized altered the life of the individual sufficient enough to give her a new direction and an unblocked avenue for moving forward. Rather than utilizing an approach that bewailed heredity or "emphasized" the mistakes made in the woman's upbringing, the positive aspects of the client were utilized to plan a shift in direction and to take the first step.

During the work with Latino women, I discovered that the work of Leona Tyler (1960) and the theory of minimum-change therapy could be pursued both in concept and in practice. Its most fundamental assumption is that there are many different ways an individual can live richly and well. Equally important is the naturalness for a person to continue to develop throughout her life in her own unique way. It may very well be unnecessary for Latino women to take on the task of changing the Latino culture now, but it is necessary to eliminate feelings of depression by taking steps toward empowering themselves to create options from which to choose courses of action.

One of the typical cases involved Rosa, a Central American, mother of two sons and common-law wife of an upper-class male from her country. Rosa had been employed in his family's business when they first met and subsequently started to live together. When the family migrated to the U.S., she came along to work as a servant in the house of her common-law husband. The situation became intolerable when the man's mother found a prospective wife for her son.

At this point, Rosa and her sons moved into a studio with a friend who was in a similar situation. In exchange for a meager monthly allowance, Rosa agreed to take her sons to visit their paternal grandmother twice a week in order to maintain her children's patrimony. She was, however, required to wait for them downstairs while the children visited with their grandmother.

Rosa came to my attention after the counselor to whom she had been assigned was unable to continue seeing her. Her file revealed that she had been in counseling for 18 months, that she complained about feeling depressed, nauseated, and generally sick. She suffered from severe headaches which she described as "dolor de celebro." Although she had been referred to various clinics for tests and x-rays, it became obvious that there was no definitive physical diagnosis for her.

After a lengthy interview, a number of facts became clear. Rosa wanted her children to continue their relationship with their grandmother in the hope that they would be treated to their advantage when they grew up. She would accept her common-law husband back, if he ever wanted to come back. She wanted to feel economically safe. She had a great desire to be taller and she felt hopeless and totally unable to change her situation.

An assessment of Rosa's educational skills revealed that with some help she might possibly be employed in an entry-level clerical position at a local bank. A program was devised that produced some short-term successes such that she began to feel confident about her ability to do clerical work. With some tutoring on test-taking, as well as on interviewing techniques, she was able to get an entry-level position at a bank. She also began to face the world with a fresh perspective. Her health improved dramatically and she began to change her appearance. She started to wear very high heels and had her hair styled, both efforts to appear taller.

In a follow-up conference a year later, Rosa reported that all was well: she and her common-law husband were seeing a lot of each other and she had had the satisfaction of rejecting her would-be mother-in-law's economic help. She was very proud of her boys' scholastic achievements and spoke of the salary raise she was about to receive, her new living accommodations, and her plans for the future.

In this case, personality reorganization was not the goal. Rather than delve into the anxieties and conflicts in which she was enmeshed, we worked to find an unblocked path to enable her to move forward and to develop her unique strengths. She was able to make a relatively minor shift in her psychological direction. A simple move *toward* self-sufficiency and *away* from a state of dependency altered her life. Rosa's world remained essentially the same: there had been no dramatic transformation of her world, but her direction and manner of coping with her reality had been altered.

The strength of this counseling approach is that more emphasis is placed on positive diagnoses. Minimal attention is paid to personality weaknesses that are controlled by society or by culture.

Only the difficulties that are actually blocking the person's movement forward are treated or, if possible, bypassed.

RECOMMENDATIONS FOR THE FUTURE

1. Government agencies must be required to collect a variety of data on Hispanics in the U.S. by subgroup, not just the three major groups included in HHANES. This would enable planning agencies to consider the needs of the diverse groups that comprise this population.
2. The youthfulness of the Latino population highlights the need for a large-scale, national health campaign for parents and children on preventive health care issues, including substance abuse. To succeed, it must have the active support of the public schools, local health-care delivery systems, and law-enforcement and judicial officials.
3. Community-based programs should be developed to address the employment, health, and mental health needs of the Latino group represented. Latino professionals should participate in the studies and in the interpretation of data that become the bases of proposed remedies. Their participation lends credibility to the efforts and increases sensitivity to the cultural needs of this population.
4. Counseling and mental health programs should consider an approach based on the psychology of development and individual differences rather than on the psychology of adjustment, recognizing that it is natural for a person to continue to develop throughout life in his or her unique way.
5. A strong effort toward changing national attitudes toward Hispanics to ones that are more positive is imperative. Changes in prevailing perceptions should minimize stresses to all involved, diminish racism, and recognize the prominent and rightful place of Hispanics in the development of this country. This effort must be established and recognized as a responsibility of those who presently influence and control the media and the education of this country. This is a worthy goal, particularly because it affects the largest minority group of the coming century and the United States as a whole.

REFERENCES

California Commission on the Status of Women (1983). An overview of minority women in the work force. *The feminization of poverty*. Sacramento: California Commission on the Status of Women.

Bachrach, L. L. (1975). *Utilization of state and county mental hospitals by Spanish Americans in 1974*. Statistical Note 116. Washington, DC: DHEW Publication No. (ADM) 75-108.

Baskin, D., Bluestone, H. & Nelson, M. (1981). Mental illness in minority women. *Journal of Clinical Psychology, 37* (3).

Becerra, R. M., Karno, M. & Escobar, J. I. (1982). *The Hispanic patient: Mental health perspectives*. New York: Grune and Stratton, Inc.

Canino, G. (1982). The Hispanic woman: Sociocultural influences on diagnoses and treatment. In M. Becerra, R. M. Karno & J. I. Escobar (Eds.), *Mental Health and Hispanic Americans*. New York: Grune and Stratton, Inc.

Castellanos, A. F. (1985, Winter). A family practice perspective. *Intercambio Feminiles, 2* (4).

Cuellos, I. (1977). The utilization of mental health facilities by Mexican Americans: A test of the underutilization hypothesis. Doctoral thesis. University of Texas at Austin.

del Portillo, C. T. (1980). The effectiveness of minimal success on positive attitude change among Latino women. Doctoral dissertation. University of San Francisco.

Garcia, K. (1980). Hispanic women: Their needs and the utilization of social services in the Mission community of San Francisco. Master of Arts Thesis. San Francisco State University.

Gibson, G. (1975). The Mexican-American woman and mental health. Paper presented at Our Lady of the Lake College, March 12, 1975.

Grossman, H. (1984). *Educating Hispanic students*. Springfield, IL: Charles C Thomas.

Ford Foundation (1984). Hispanics: Challenges and opportunities. Paper.

Heckler, M. M. (1985, winter). Hispanic health issues and government. *Intercambio Feminiles, 2* (4).

Higher education. *Wall Street Journal*, September 23, 1986.

Llanes, J. (1975). Latina self-concept. Paper presented before the Puerto Rican Organization for Women (PROW), San Francisco, California, March, 1975.

Miranda, M. R. (Ed.) (1986). *Psychotherapy with the Spanish-speaking: Issues in research and services delivery*. Monograph No. 3. Los Angeles: University of California, Spanish-Speaking Mental Health Research Center.

Melville, M. B. (Ed.) (1980). *Twice a minority*. St. Louis: The C. V. Mosby Co.

Newton, F. C., Olmedo, E. L. & Padilla, A. M. (1982). *Hispanic mental health research*. Berkeley: University of California Press.

Pietro, J. (1985, winter). What is government's responsibility in health promotion and care for Hispanic women? *Intercambio Feminiles, 2* (4).

Rendon, L. (1975). *Clinical re-socialization of women: A case study*. Masters of Arts Thesis. San Francisco State University.

Rogler, L. H. et al. (1983). *A conceptual framework for mental health research on Hispanic populations*. Monograph No. 10. New York: Fordham University, Hispanic Research Center.

Sowell, T. (1983). *The economics and politics of race*. New York: William Morrow & Co., Inc.

Special Populations Sub-Task Panel on Mental Health of Hispanic Americans (1978). *Report to the president's commission on mental health*. Los Angeles: University of California, Spanish-speaking Mental Health Research Center.

Taylor, P. (1984). Hispanic Americans haven't found their pot of gold. *The Washington Post*. National Weekly Edition, May 28, 1984.

The National School Public Relations Association (1986, July). Hispanic gaps persists. *Education U.S.A.*, *28* (47).

Torres-Matrullo, C. (1982). Cognitive therapy of depressive disorders in the Puerto Rican female. In R. M. Becerra, M. Karno, & J. I. Escobar (Eds.), *Mental Health and Hispanic Americans*. New York: Grune and Stratton, Inc.

Tyler, L. (1960). Minimum-change therapy. *Personnel & Guidance Journal. 38*.

Ullman, L. P. & Krasner, L. (1975). *A psychological approach to abnormal behavior*. Englewoods Cliffs, NJ: Prentice Hall, Inc.

U. S. Bureau of the Census (1982). Persons of Spanish origin by state: 1980. *Supplementary Report*. PC 80-S1-7.

U. S. Bureau of the Census (1985, December). *Population reports*. Series P-20, No. 403.

U. S. Department of Health and Human Services (1985). *Plan and operation of Hispanic health and nutrition examination survey. 1982-84*. Vital and Health Statistics Series 1, No. 19, DHHS Pub. No. (PHS) 85-1321.

A Social Essay
on Special Issues
Facing Poor Women of Color

Ruth H. Gordon-Bradshaw, PhD

SUMMARY. Race, gender, and socioeconomic status place poor women of color in triple jeopardy for subservience. Racism, sexism, impoverishment, and discrimination in a variety of services serve to deny poor women of color the opportunities in education, occupations, income, and health services that are afforded other groups in this country. This paper shows that the fight for civil rights is also one for preventive and quality, accessible and comprehensive care for those who suffer most: poor women of color, and that until this nation is purged of these egregious and reprehensible forces, the goal of a true democracy will continue to elude us.

INTRODUCTION

At least three-fourths of the world's population is distributed among people of color—broadly classified as nonwhite, and includingthose designated as "minority": Blacks, Hispanics, Native Americans, Asians, and Alaskans/Pacific Islanders. Women in this group outnumber men and make up approximately one-half of the world's population. In the United States, despite comprising 51 percent of the population, women are treated as a "minority" (Shahanish, 1985; Welsing, 1970). The imposed "minority" status of women in general places poor women of color in triple jeopardy for subservience by virtue of their race, gender, and socioeconomic status (Christmas, 1984).

Ruth H. Gordon-Bradshaw is President, Gordshaw Professional Health and Development Services, Inc., 301 East Riding Road, Montgomery, AL 36116.

White men have arrogated to themselves the right to rule — the power component of the "majority status." Such a structure affords preferential treatment in education, jobs, and control over other societal institutions for those of the "ruling class" and inequality and subjugation for women of color. It is described in the *Fourth World Manifesto* thusly:

> American society is one of structured social inequality, in which there is an unequal distribution of rewards based on gender, race and class difference. (Carmen, Russo & Miller, 1981)

Racism, sexism, prejudice, discrimination, poverty, poor health, and low educational achievement seriously compromise the quality of life for a significant segment of U.S. society. While sexism is the economic exploitation and social condemnation of members of one gender by others, racism is utilized by groups to overcome psychological and social insecurities at the expense of other groups. The predominant form of racism in the United States is a delusion arising from the false premise that white skin color presumes an overall, generalized, and unrivaled superiority (Pierce, 1975). A society such as that in the United States may promote and reward racism to enable some members to experience a sense of personal adequacy and security at the expense of other members. If freedom and equality are true goals, racism, sexism, and other forms of discrimination must be purged from this nation, an effort requiring a large-scale local, state, and national commitment and preventive measures to disallow its resurgence.

Despite a system of rhetorical democracy and a land of plenty, the dreams of those who comprise America's poor are too often dashed and replaced with a life of impoverishment. Reflecting on the words of Victor Hugo:

> So long as there shall exist, by virtue of law and custom, a social damnation artificially creating hells in the midst of civilization, and complicating the Divine destiny with a fatality which is human, so long as three great problems are not solved, the degradation of man through poverty, the

ruin of women through hunger, and the crippling of children through ignorance . . . so long as such wretchedness exists on earth, papers like this must be written.

Special issues related to laws and customs stemming from gender, race, and class pose barriers to a variety of social, economic, and health services. In this paper several social indicators of equality—education, living environment, employment and income, poverty, and health—are examined to assess the at-risk status of poor women of color. The World Health Organization's definition of health as a state of positive well-being—physical, mental, social, and spiritual, and not merely the absence of disease—underlies the concept of health used throughout this discussion. Health problems, on the other hand, undermine this state of well-being and serve to keep women of color from living longer and better lives.

EDUCATION

It is generally held that the nature of one's schooling partly determines the kind of jobs held, the amount of money earned, and one's lifelong socioeconomic status. Because of these factors and the belief in an informed citizenry, education in this country has developed as a right for all children. Yet, all children do not enjoy the benefits of this right. Poor young women of color today, like their sisters before them, have experienced serious inequities in schooling and educational opportunities.

More than 40 percent of American Indian/Alaskan Native females in 1960 were at least two years behind the schooling progress of their peers. The gap increased from 1970 to 1976, when it began to narrow. At that time, however, 25 percent or more American Indian/Alaskan Native, Mexican American, and Puerto Rican females were still two years behind in the grade-level skills expected for students of their ages.

As important as the skills they fail to develop, those who fall behind in school also become more likely to drop out. Evidence suggests that among the predictors of dropping out is being two or more years behind grade level; girls within this group are most likely to become pregnant. Data from the High School and Beyond studies show that youth from households with low-income, low-skill wage earners, and limited educational opportunities drop out at a rate three times that for those from the highest end of the socioeconomic scale (22 percent vs. 7 percent). This is true particularly for poor women of color, and it is happening far too frequently.

While more females today are graduating from high school than in the past, the dropout rate increases as they ascend the educational ladder as does the gap in high school completion between whites and nonwhites. Evidence of disadvantaged background becomes more obvious and more severe as individuals reach the critical teenage years. By the time of entrance into secondary schools, thousands of Black and Hispanic fourteen- to seventeen-year-olds already have dropped out or are at risk of dropping out. In the major cities of this country, where large segments of this population reside, dropout rates for Black and Hispanic females frequently exceed 40 percent.

Whatever success that may have been realized in stemming high school dropout rates in the past is being eroded by adolescent mothers who drop out of school and enter into a cycle of poverty with lifelong consequences (U.N. Decade for Women, 1985). Adolescents who are behind in grade-level performance or who lack basic skills are at risk of early parenthood. According to the Children's Defense Fund (1986), a National Labor Survey of sixteen- to seventeen-year-olds revealed that girls who fell in the bottom quartile on basic skills tests were five times more likely to become mothers than those girls who obtained average scores. In addition, poor youth, whether Black, Hispanic, or white, are three to four times more likely to become unwed parents than their advantaged peers. And, young mothers are more likely than their peers to drop out of school (Children's Defense Fund, 1986).

If a poor female student of color remains in school, she is typically tracked in vocational, general, or special education programs, without consideration of her ability or potential. Moreover, poor students of color with physical and mental health disabilities are likely to go without the educational support that would enable them to develop their potential, adversely affecting their academic performance and school attendance (Children's Defense Fund, 1986). The communities in which poor female students of color reside often offer few or no programs of support or challenge, or other activities that would assist these youth.

Those who leave high school without a diploma experience more difficulty in obtaining the types of jobs and incomes than those who have completed their high school education. Numerous social indices attest to measures of success in life when a quality educational experience has been acquired. It is unreasonable to expect success in life when those opportunities are denied. The link between schooling and job opportunity is just too critical. Corrective action measures must be instituted to retain female students of color in high school, to enhance their development, and to facilitate their future productivity (Children's Defense Fund, 1986).

Female students of color who manage to graduate from high school and to enroll in higher education programs are most frequently clustered in lower-cost two-year colleges. Yet, their presence on college campuses of all types is declining. Despite dramatic improvements in high school completion rates for Blacks over the last two decades, college attendance and completion rates have declined for Blacks since 1975, and the data on Blacks and Hispanics in colleges compared to whites show that the gap has widened (The College Board, 1985).

To reverse this trend in declining college completion, retention programs with specific characteristics are required. Recommendations for retaining poor students of color in colleges include a variety of strategies: high levels of institutional commitment to integrate retention efforts into the college's mission, comprehensive services, dedicated staff and strong faculty support, participation in supportive services programs without stigma, role models and mentors, and collection of data in order to monitor academic progress (Educational Testing Service, 1985).

LIVING ENVIRONMENT

Poverty is a pervasive theme in the lives of poor women of color. While poverty is primarily assessed by income measures, it is also a social condition apparent by such indicators as housing, schooling, nutrition, and medical care. It affords an unequal distribution of means and privileges. It is a condition in which the essence is inequality.

Poor women of color are concentrated in inner cities across the nation. Because of their limited financial resources, they typically have no choice but to live in housing and environments that increase their vulnerability to hazards and disease. The data in Table 1 illustrate this point. Higher rates of morbidity and mortality from accidental injuries such as asphyxiation resulting from faulty heaters and house fires may be attributed to poor living conditions in low-income housing areas of inner cities. In the urban environment, poor women of color are also likely exposed to numerous environmental hazards: pollution, noise, substandard and overcrowded housing, homicide and crime, poor nutrition, and unsanitary living conditions, with the attendant problems of stress stemming from each of these factors (Heckler, 1986).

A classic picture of environmental hazards poor women often face is provided by Bullough and Bullough (1982). The authors recount an anecdote that describes how rats mutilated and killed an infant in a substandard housing project in a major urban city. Issues such as public transportation, an inadequate health care delivery system, housing discrimination because of ethnicity and marital status, child care, and public administrative inertia reflect the conflicting and patchwork public policies relative to the poor and the overwhelming problems of the living environment. The diminishing number of housing units available to low-income families also leads to an increasing number of women and children among the homeless.

EMPLOYMENT AND INCOME

While many have migrated to cities from rural areas in search of employment, opportunities to move out of poverty are limited (Heckler, 1986). In 1982, the unemployment rate for Blacks was reported at 18.9 percent, more than double the rate for whites. These official rates, however, underestimate the depth of the problem as they do not include discouraged workers who have abandoned their search for a job.

Table 1

Age-Adjusted Death Rates by Selected Cause, Race

and Sex in the United States, 1980

(Rate per 100,000 Population)

	Black Male	White Male	Relative Risk	Black Female	White Female	Relative Risk
Total Deaths						
(All Causes)	1,112.8	745.3	1.5	631.1	411.1	1.5
Heart Disease	327.3	277.5	1.2	201.1	134.6	1.5
Stroke	77.5	41.9	1.9	61.7	35.2	1.8
Cancer	229.9	160.5	1.4	129.7	107.7	1.2
Infant Mortality	2,586.7	1,230.3	2.1	2,123.7	962.5	2.2
Homicide	71.9	10.9	6.6	13.7	3.2	4.3
Accidents	82.0	62.3	1.3	25.1	21.4	1.2
Cirrhosis	30.6	15.7	2.0	14.4	7.0	2.1
Diabetes	17.7	9.5	1.9	22.1	8.7	2.5

SOURCE: NCHS, Health: United States, 1983, Tables 9 and 15.

For those who are able to acquire employment, the workplace represents another source of hazards to physical well-being (see Stellman, this issue). Employment in positions substantially lower on the occupational ladder exposes poor women to greater risks from occupational hazards such as physical and mental stressors, and toxic substances (Children's Defense Fund, 1986).

These jobs also pay low wages. Black family median income in 1982 was only 55 percent of that reported for whites: $13,598 vs. $24,603 (The College Board, 1985). Blacks and other persons of color have lost ground economically, both in relative and absolute terms. And for low-income women of color, the jobs held offer few, if any opportunities for advancement.

Table 2 presents the distribution of minority groups by type of occupation and the ratio of nonminority to minority group individuals in these jobs. These data show that in relation to whites, fewer Blacks, Asians, Native Americans, and Hispanics are represented in white-collar occupations. Because of the differences in the types of jobs held, additional years of schooling between elementary school and college do not net consistent nor commensurate gains in employability for Blacks in the same way that they do for whites.

It has been suggested that a discriminatory outcome of women's increased labor force participation in the 1970s may have been to limit women to occupations below their skill levels (U.S. Commission on Civil Rights, 1978). It is not uncommon for women (and men) of color to demonstrate greater skill or more educational accomplishments — to be overqualified — in order to obtain employment. Even in a labor market where the match between peoples' qualifications and their jobs supposedly is free from racial or gender bias, a disproportionately high number of minority persons surpass the stated requirements for their occupations (U.S. Commission on Civil Rights, 1978).

It is generally assumed that remaining in school increases a person's chances for better jobs and higher salaries. Are the rewards for schooling equivalent for women of color? Absolutely not, according to the U.S. Commission on Civil Rights (1978). Even though educational attainment is linked to earning power, persons in different demographic groups with the same educational preparation do not earn the same income. Women of color

Table 2

Occupational Distribution of Minority Groups

Ratio of Nonminority to Minority*

Occupation	Black		Asian		Native American		Hispanic	
Sex:	M	F	M	F	M	F	M	F
White Collar	1.39	1.59	1.03	.96	1.50	2.04	4.70	--
Blue Collar	.77	.85	.88	1.42	.68	.77	1.54	--
Farm	1.56	1.08	1.20	1.03	.78	.66	--	--
Service	.56	.49	1.03	.35	.57	.57	.13	--
Employed	1.08	1.07	1.90	1.39	2.95	1.82	--	--

SOURCE: Department of Commerce: A Statistical Analysis. Women in the United States. Series P-23, No. 100. Washington, D.C.

*Represents the ratio of nonminority to minority. For example, 39 percent more nonminority males are in white collar occupations than Black males.

who do manage to overcome the obstacles to obtain a college education, for example, find their financial rewards significantly lower than those of men with the same educational backgrounds. In fact, no college-educated group of women earned as much as 70 percent of the average income of white males in 1975 (U.S. Commission on Civil Rights, 1978) (see Table 3).

Women of color are most likely to be unemployed or employed in jobs less valued by society, and segregated from whites in the types of jobs they hold. As the data above show, the distribution of jobs remains skewed to the detriment of women of color. Their overrepresentation in jobs and occupations in which private pension funds and similar benefits are unavailable tend to increase the reliance of women of color on Social Security and public welfare (Children's Defense Fund, 1986; Heckler, 1986). Such work conditions can only foster protracted poverty in the advanced years, when there is an increased demand for benefits such as health care services. This places aged women of color at special risk.

The elderly minority population is growing faster than that for whites according to the American Association of Retired Persons News Bulletin (October 1986). This trend is expected to continue and is projected to comprise approximately 20 percent of the 65 and older age cohort by the year 2050. Older women of color are more likely to live alone or to live in or near poverty. Age and health status are often assumed to be causal factors of impoverishment (see Grau, this volume). Although a diminished income and mounting expenses are mitigating factors, many aged poor women of color were always poor. Being aged, poor, and female has been one description of triple jeopardy. Being of color greatly compounds an already difficult status.

POVERTY

Women of color fall at the bottom of the economic ladder (see Wilson, this volume). They find themselves poor despite their efforts to earn an adequate income to provide for their basic needs. High unemployment, low wages, and long hours of work under adverse conditions make their struggle for survival even

Table 3

Selected Social Characteristics of Women of Color

Racial Group	Percent of Female in Workforce	Schooling		Median Annual Income[a]	Female Headed Household[d]	Unemployment Rate
		H.S.	College			(1982)
Blacks	same as white women	79%	13%	$13,270	37.7%	18.9%
Hispanics	49%	58%	10%	16,228	23.0%	13.8%[b]
Asian/ Pacific Islanders	58%	75%	33%	22,713[c]	11.0%	4.7%
Native Americans	48%	31%	7%	15,900	25.0%	13.0%

SOURCE: Report of the Secretary's Task Force on Black and Minority Health, DHHS, August, 1985.

a. One out of every 3 Blacks, Hispanics and Native Americans (34%) lived below the poverty level in 1981.

b. Among Puerto Rican families, the rate of 40%.

c. According to 1980 Census, the median income is consistently rising.

d. Their children suffer a much higher rate of poverty (54 percent in 1984) than other children according to Children Defense Fund 1987 Budget Analysis.

more difficult. Against seemingly unsurmountable odds, they are not able to earn the required income to pull themselves and their children out of poverty.

Full-time employment at minimum wage salaries will not prevent these families from winding up in poverty. One of the main contributing factors is the stagnation of the minimum wage. In the past, the minimum wage kept up with inflation, but under the current federal administration it has remained at the same level (see Table 4). Thus families where the household head works full-time at the hourly minimum wage fall deeper into poverty. A women holding a job paying a minimum-wage salary in 1986 is taking home less than four-fifths of what she earned in 1980. By comparing the declining value of the minimum wage to the inflation-tied rise in poverty levels, many families have been pushed into poverty.

HEALTH

It is a paradox that the United States can achieve such greatness in science, technology, and the health of the overall population, but continues to disenfranchise people of color by fostering disparities in health care. Improvements in the overall health of U.S. citizens and advancements in medical science have not remedied the serious inequities in the health care system and health status for the most vulnerable – Blacks, Hispanics, Native Americans and Asian/Pacific Islanders (Heckler, 1986).

Poverty reaps havoc on people of color because of their limited resources and lack of access to health care, and lends credence to the adage that "those who suffer most get the least." Data reported by the Department of Health and Human Services' Task Force on Black and Minority Health for the period 1979 to 1981 identified six causes of death that account for 80 percent of the mortality among Blacks and other people of color. These include: cancer, cardiovascular disease and stroke, chemical dependency, measured by deaths due to cirrhosis, diabetes, homicide and accidents (unintentional injuries), and infant mortality.

The quantification of health problems can be found in actuarial tables and in social equality indicators depicting increased mor-

Table 4

Minimum Wage and Income

Year	Hourly Minimum Wage	Annual Earnings for 2,000 Hours' Work (50 Weeks of 40 Hours	Poverty Level (3 Persons)	Full-Time Minimum Wage Earnings As Percent of Poverty Level for 3
1964	$1.25	$2,500	$2,413	103.6%
1969	1.60	3,200	2,924	109.4
1974	2.00	4,000	3,936	101.6
1979	2.90	5,800	5,784	100.3
1980	3.10	6,200	6,565	94.4
1981	3.35	6,700	7,250	92.4
1982	3.35	6,700	7,693	87.1
1983	3.35	6,700	7,938	84.4
1984	3.35	6,700	8,277	80.9
1985	3.35	6,700	8,589 (est.)	78.0
1986	3.35	6,700	8,934 (est.)	75.0

Source: Children Defense Fund: Analysis of FY 1987 Budget for Children.

tality, morbidity, and vulnerability to illness. The limited access to affordable health care creates the dilemma that individuals delay seeking medical attention and are diagnosed at much later stages of illness, thereby drastically increasing the likelihood that the prognosis will be poor (American Cancer Society, 1983). Recent mortality data support this point. Forty-two percent, or about 59,000 of the 240,000 deaths experienced by Blacks each year, would not have occurred had Blacks experienced the same age-sex rates as whites. These are "excess deaths." Sixty thousand more people of color than whites die each year from the causes listed above because of significant inequities in health care systems (Hackett, 1985; Heckler, 1986), and because certain age and racial groups experience a higher rate of death than others because of health problems specific to that group. For Black males and females combined, for example, excess deaths accounted for 47 percent of the total annual deaths in those age 45 years and younger, and for 42 percent of the deaths in those aged 70 years and under. While the data for Asians are more promising, the data for Native American and Hispanics are no more encouraging (Heckler, 1986).

Black women of childbearing age are four times more likely to die in childbirth, and their children are three times as likely as white children to become a postneonatal mortality statistic. These problems are attributed to poverty. Inadequate perinatal care, poor nutrition (e.g., high salt intake and limited ingestion of dairy products because of lactose intolerances), inability to afford vitamin and mineral supplements, and the marked prevalence of obesity among Black women place them at risk during the perinatal period. Early perinatal care and improvements in the general living environment and dietary practices of poor women may be the initial, important steps in improving their health status (National Black Women's Health Project, 1986).

Poor children are three times less likely than nonpoor children to have adequate health insurance for the entire year. The problems associated with access to health care are compounded as 80 percent of these children are afflicted with one or more untreated medical conditions (Children's Defense Fund, 1986). In infancy and childhood, poor nutrition and health can negatively affect cognitive development and can increase the possibilities for developmental disabilities and learning disorders. During child-hood and adolescent periods, untreated visual, hearing, dental, and mental health problems are examples of general poor health and can contribute to poor academic performance and poor school attendance (Children's Defense Fund, 1986). In addition, increases in adolescent suicides exemplify the hopelessness and despair. Black female and Native American teenage suicides ex-ceed those of whites.

These factors suggest that the fight for civil rights is also one for preventive and quality, accessible and comprehensive care for those who suffer most—poor women of color. Financial and cultural barriers to services too often negatively influence their lives. This is also evidence that poor women of color pay a hefty price for their triple minority status. In a true democratic society, the knowledge and practices leading to a better health standard and prolonged life in one sector of society must be shared among all citizens.

CONCLUDING REMARKS

For poor women of color, the response to inequity and depri-vation is a quest for power, control, and self-acquisition. The response to resistance to equality is further alienation, rejection, and conflict. We cannot continue to be politically tyrannized, socially minimized, economically ignored, and victims of poor nutrition, sterilization and experimentation, and a variety of other preventable and treatable conditions. A genuine commit-ment to social change is *action* and self-empowerment. Finally, I remind all my sisters that we may have come to this country in different boats and for different reasons but if you are poor, we are now in the same boat.

RECOMMENDATIONS

To poor women of color:

— Create dissatisfaction in being violated, docile, and accept-ing adults: demand full equality; show an unwillingness to remain uneducated, dependent, hopeless, earning lower incomes, living in substandard conditions, and experiencing poor health. To do otherwise is to supply a rationale for contempt.

— Develop self-confidence for enhancing trust of each other, and then work to unite over common concerns. Without unification, the powerless become even more powerless.

— Develop coalitions among women of color to form businesses to create meaningful jobs for us and our children.

— Lobby for tax incentives for organizations to employ "qualifiable women," qualify them, and prepare a career advancement plan in nontraditional occupations.

To state and federal policymakers:

— Raise child care to a national priority with an adequate federal subsidy. Provide tax incentives to employers who provide child care.

— Restructure human service programs and providers to foster independency by providing immediate assistance with a plan for personal growth, an emphasis on health promotion and disease prevention throughout the life cycle, and a concern for the quality of life for clients. Require these programs to acknowledge the validity and to integrate the cultural experiences of Blacks, Hispanics, Native Americans and Alaskan/Pacific Islanders, and particularly women, in designing services and interacting with clients.

— Provide school-based health services, including dental, mental health and formal family life education programs, and day care facilities for teenage parents.

— Sponsor federal funding for community-based family crisis teams accessible by hotline and mobile units available 24 hours daily for crisis intervention in rape, family violence, and suicide.

— Revitalize affirmative action for eradication of institutionalized racism and sexism.

— Preserve the right to quality health care for all citizens by making it affordable, accessible, acceptable, and comprehensive.

— Revise the education/socialization process to eliminate gender- and race-based role ascriptions so each person may develop to her/his maximum potential.
— Lobby for passage of the Equal Rights Amendment.

REFERENCES

American Cancer Society (1983). *Cancer facts and figures for minority Americans.*
Bullough, V. & Bullough, B. (1982). *Health care for the other Americans.* New York: Appleton Century-Crofts.
Carmen, E. H., Russo, N. F. & Miller, J. B. (1981). Inequality and women's mental health: An overview. *American Journal of Psychiatry, 138,* 1319-1330.
Children's Defense Fund (1986). *An analysis of the FY 1987 federal budget and children.* Washington, D.C.: Children's Defense Fund.
Christmas, J. (1984): Black women and health care. *Spelman Message, 100,* (1).
College Board, The (1985). *Equality and excellence: The educational status of black Americans.* New York: College Entrance Examination Board.
Fourth World Manifesto, January 13, 1971.
Hackett, D. (1985, December). The greeks. *Crisis.* 75th anniversary issue: 51-52.
Heckler, M. M. (1986). *Report of the secretary's task force on black and minority health.* Washington, DC: U.S. Department of Health and Human Services.
Hugo, V. In H. P. Miller (1966), *Poverty: American style.* Belmont, CA: Wadsworth.
National Black Women's Health Project (1986). *Open your life.* Atlanta, GA.
Pierce, C. M. (1974). Psychiatric problems of the black minority. In G. Caplan (Ed.), *American Handbook of Psychiatry* (2nd.). New York: Basic Books.
Shahanish, L. R. (1985). Mexico to Copenhagen to Nairobi: An irresistible momentum. *U.N. Chronicle. XXII* (ii).
U.N. Decade for Women Status Report. (1985, June). American black women: Their influence on the American economy—A current status of America's first female work force. Proceedings of Wingspread Conference, Atlanta, Georgia.
U.S. Commission on Civil Rights (1978). *Social indicators of equality for minorities and women.* Washington, DC.
Welsing, F. C. (1970). *The cross theory of color.* Washington, DC.